My Enemy, My Friend

The touching and inspirational true story of how a young girl used her positive attitude to overcome debilitating Arthritis

By Lauren Vaknine

Acknowledgements

There are so many people whom I would like to thank for helping me, not only during the process of writing and creating this book, but also those who have helped me throughout my life.

The doctors: Dr Keat, Dr Pavesio, Dr Fisher, Dr Roniger, Dr Khan, Ady Shanan, Lubina Mohamed and Trish Raven. Also the Royal London Hospital for Integrated Medicine.

My wonderful friends, what would life be without the family we choose for ourselves? Thank you for your continued support.

Team Creative! Brooke Berlyn, Stevie Sollinger, Nicole Springer and everyone at Lightning Source.

A huge thanks also goes out to others who helped along the journey in all sorts of ways, financial and other: Rosi and David Kalev, Jonny Matthews, Shirley Harris and Susan Kogan.

Most importantly, my family. The ones who love unconditionally and stay beside me even when I am the least desirable person to be around. Mum, Aba, Ilana and the angel who is my husband, Daniel. Thank you will never be enough.

Lastly, a thank you to those in spirit who continually inspire me: Nanny, Poppa, Jake and the spirit force that holds us all together.

This book is dedicated to my mother.

Mummy, anything I have achieved so far is because of you. Anything I will achieve in the future is for you.

My strength, my saviour, my best friend.

Love Dotty

The block of granite which is an obstacle in the pathway of the weak, becomes a stepping stone in the pathway of the strong.

Thomas Carlyle

Prologue

The First Diagnosis

"Come on darling, go back in the circle and join the other girls."
"But I don't like ballet, Mummy. I don't want to do it any more."

The great thing about children is that they have the sort of resilience that adults cannot understand. If they have a certain pain, they believe that this is normal and that everyone feels this in their bodies because they have nothing to compare it with. This is why, when I was four years old and I walked out of the circle of aspiring ballerinas at my local ballet class, I couldn't tell my mum that it hurt my knees and ankles too much to reach those tough ballet positions. I just assumed that I didn't like ballet. It was only about 15 years later, in an attempt to find answers in order to try and heal myself, that the pieces of the puzzle started to fit together and a lot of things started to make sense about my childhood.

I will start from the beginning to give you a clearer picture: a few months before my second birthday, my parents noticed swelling around my ankles. They took me to the GP, who did not recognise the cause, and he referred me to the Royal National Orthopaedic Hospital, a world class hospital which was quite conveniently situated not five minutes from where we lived. A series of doctors examined me, but no one could come to any real conclusions about the problem as the swelling was not going down and was now spreading to my knees. I was booked in for a biopsy. I had to stay in the children's ward overnight and I have a vague memory of that ward. Although I was very young – twenty-three months to be precise – there are some events that, somehow, I still remember.

There were not many patients in the ward and most children had at least one of their parents with them. There was a waiting room attached to the ward with a dirty fish tank in it and one of the children in a bed near me was the daughter of one of the doctors – I'm still not quite sure what she was doing there. She was eating chocolate mousse from a plastic pot with her hands and I remember thinking that the smell of it was rancid.

I don't remember being scared or worried, but I think I was too young to know what was going on. Also, I had my parents with me the whole time, which makes a young child feel secure even at the worst of times.

The next morning, the paediatrician came to see me before my biopsy. He took one look at me and told my parents that I didn't need a biopsy. "She has Stills Disease," he said. Translated into words that my parents could understand, this doctor whom we never saw again, diagnosed me with Juvenile Arthritis, or Juvenile Idiopathic Arthritis as it was then known, idiopathic meaning a condition with no defined cause. It really did have no defined cause, or so we thought at the time. Doctors still tend to believe that it has no defined cause but luckily for me, I now have more information and reject this idea. We were told that it had stemmed from a virus I had had a few months before, but the illness had probably been dormant in my body since I was born – the virus was the catalyst that triggered it. Or so we thought. I speak about this and explain it in more depth right at the end of the book.

My mother often talked about all the thoughts that went through her head when the doctor gave his diagnosis: 'Oh my God, what the hell is that now??' And, of course, the worry didn't go away when they were told that this was arthritis.

Like most people, my parents assumed that arthritis only affects the elderly. It does, in fact, affect about one in every 10,000 children. Considering how small a percentage this is, how did it come to pass that one day I had a virus and the next, arthritis, which would essentially shape the rest of my life? I have my theories (again, at the end of the book) but I have never asked 'why me?', because I have come to learn that everything in this life happens for a reason, even if that reason is not clear to us (or our poor parents) at the time.

After I was diagnosed, I was referred to the Rheumatology Department at Northwick Park Hospital in Harrow, London, under Dr. Barbara Ansell who, at the time, was one of the most respected figures in the field of childhood arthritis. I remember that clinic so vividly. Although it is now a podiatry clinic, I have walked past there many times over the years when I have been in the hospital and remember how it used to be – the smells, the people, the doctors. There must have been a recurring theme of fish tanks in hospitals, as this one had a huge tank against the wall of the waiting area. I always remember looking forward to going there just to see the fish. Maybe it was because in 1986 they didn't have computer games in hospitals to keep children occupied, just fish tanks, books and a blue or red plastic box full of donated toys and games, like the trusted old Etch-A-Sketch and the Bluebird Big Yellow Teapot.

Dr. Ansell assessed me then asked my parents why I was so short for my age. "She's actually way above average height for her age," Mum said. "She's not even two yet." "Oh I am sorry," said Dr Ansell. "She speaks so fluently, I thought she was at least four!" Mum said I spoke at two years old better than most four year olds spoke, completely fluently in both English and Hebrew, and was able not only to put sentences together but also to converse.

I don't really remember Dr. Ansell, though I have read a lot about her and the research she has done into Juvenile Arthritis over the years. It is strange the things that children remember. My parents often tell me about events that I don't remember happening, such as, I suppose, meeting such a prominent figure as Dr. Ansell, but I do remember my first day at nursery.

There were four classes, two for older children and two for the younger ones. I was in the Cygnets and would later move up to the Swans. I remember hearing the names of children being called out, names I had never heard before, like Sophie, and some of these children, including Sophie, are still close friends of mine today. I remember being given a cup of orange squash and a biscuit as a mid-morning snack, which I found quite strange as I didn't think that the two went together very well – not to mention that orange squash couldn't have been the healthiest option – and I even recall what some of the rooms in the building looked like.

Maybe we block out certain things, as children, that do not seem relevant. I know that I do have both good and bad memories from my childhood and from growing up with arthritis. However, I have now come to realise that my misfortune was probably harder for my parents than it ever was for me, as they remember every detail, every hospital, every diagnosis and every bad memory, and these will be forever engraved on their minds. So I hope that what follows in this book will not only help the people who are themselves going through the agony of an illness, whether it be physical or emotional, but also their families – the ones who cannot block out the memories, the ones who do not forget.

Lauren Vaknine
February 2010

Chapter 1

The Second Diagnosis

Following the first diagnosis, my life continued in as normal a way as possible. The month after I was diagnosed, I celebrated my second birthday at home with a Postman Pat birthday cake, specially made by the quaint little cake shop on Edgware high street that all the mums got their kids' cakes from and was as busy as an ice cream hut on a hot day but for some reason still closed down during some point in my childhood. It was quite a big party considering it was at home. I think my parents were over-compensating for something over which they had no control.

My mum, what can I say about my mum to give her the credit she so rightly deserves? As you read on you'll see she doesn't need me to give her credit, she did it all for herself. She is and always was a strong woman. Emotionally, she was superman. She was always quite pretty, my mum, with dark, almost shoulder-length hair. She has a rather warped sense of humour which most find funny, others – namely fourteen year old daughters – tend to find it embarrassing. But she is and always will be the life and soul of the party and the one person that everyone turns to for advice. She is compassionate yet tough at the same time, the best kind of person to seek advice from.

After the diagnosis, she did everything in her power to make our situation better. She never cried (not in front of me, anyway) and she always tried to find ways to keep me happy.

So my Dad, the tough, strong, tall, muscly former-Israeli army man, known to me as Aba (Hebrew for Dad), how did he deal with the diagnosis and consequences that resulted from it? All I can say – and his younger self would probably wince at the thought – is that he simply defied all the aforementioned adjectives describing his attributes when it came to my illness. He just couldn't deal with it, and the emotions that had been buried away so deep for most of his life, came rushing to the surface when he saw me in pain.

Aba was born in Casablanca, Morocco, and moved to Israel at the age of twenty. He is now seventy but his daily trips to the gym have kept him looking, and feeling, young. He is very tall and has huge, almost reptile-like protruding blue eyes that look kind when he is smiling but scary when he is angry.

My maternal grandparents lived five minutes from us, but they'd only moved there from the East End shortly before I was diagnosed. They were your typical East End Jews; my poppa had spent his entire life working in a tobacco factory and Nanny raised the kids. They didn't have much but were content with pie and mash on a Saturday and a cup of cockles every so often. They took the news especially badly and spent much time trying to work out why it had happened. But, there were no answers and I was inordinately unaware of what was going on.

We were told that there was a strong chance that the arthritis could burn itself out by the time I reached adolescence, or even before, and I think my family firmly held onto that hope. At two years old, the only signs of my arthritis were swollen knees and ankles. No one knew if I was in pain or whether the condition would always stay as stable as it was then. There were no answers as to where this was going and I suppose this must have been the hardest aspect for my family. When you don't know what to expect, you don't know how best to move forward, and this is where bad decisions are often made regarding treatment options.

There was no Internet in those days so it wasn't easy to research the condition and find answers. We had to rely on what the doctors told us and I think my family found this very difficult. Mum kept thinking that there must be more to it, the doctors couldn't possibly know everything. That revelation has been my saviour. That, and the fact that she took herself to the library and only emerged three days later, when she felt she had finally absorbed enough information to make a decision, and the most significant thing she learned was that drugs have side effects. Bad ones.

But there was another blow to come.

There is a condition connected to JRA (JRA stands for Juvenile Rheumatoid Arthritis, even though some still call it JIA (idiopathic) and I will refer to it as this many times in this book), which affects the eyes. Called uveitis, it causes inflammation in the anterior chamber of the eye (the iris). For reasons still unbeknown to doctors after much research, there is a pretty high chance – as much as 20% - that children with JRA will develop uveitis. Children with pauciarticular arthritis – those with four or fewer joints affected within the first six months – are at a much higher risk of developing uveitis, and it is also more common in girls. Basically, I was the perfect candidate. Because of this, I was referred to an ophthalmologist and was tested every few months. By my third birthday, I had been diagnosed with uveitis.

Again, it was one of those things that I didn't really understand. Hospitals became a way of life and so I saw this as the norm, not really understanding the fact that not every three year-old went through this. The good news was that I only had it in one eye, my right eye, and the doctors advised us that it was unlikely to develop in both eyes. Of course, anything was possible, so I was monitored through monthly check-ups.

Uveitis can usually be controlled by steroid eye drops which reduce the inflammation in the eye and although my parents had decided against oral steroids for the joints, they didn't think it was an option to play around when it came to the eye. I was given two types of eye drops; Maxidex and Mydricacyl, medically known as Dexamethasone and Tropicamide and known to me as 'the white one and the red one', due to the colours of their lids. All I knew was that the one with the white lid was to be taken a few times during the day and the one with the red lid I took before I went to bed, and that it stung a lot. Sometimes I had to use one red one in the morning too, which I didn't like as it made my eye go very blurry. This was because the red one was a dilating eye drop and, although my eyes were not being tested every day, it was used to relax the muscles in the eye. To be honest, I still don't know exactly what this achieved, and there were many other processes that took place, or medications that I took, that I never really knew the reasoning behind. But these things became a way of life and I never felt the need to question them.

From when I was diagnosed, I was under a world-renowned ophthalmologist, Dr. Elizabeth Graham. I always saw her as being quite posh, as she was extremely well spoken. She had mousy blonde hair in a long bob with a side parting, a hairstyle that never changed for as long as I knew her. She never seemed to age or change. She had two children, Alice and George, which I thought were very posh names indeed. Yet again, I find it strange that I remember such details as my ophthalmologist's childrens' names, yet I still don't really know what the eye drops I had been taking for twenty-seven years of my life achieved. (Well, I now know that they achieved more harm than good, but more of that later.) I suppose that is how children operate. I didn't care for the details of the ingredients in the medications I was given, but I did wish to form some sort of bond with the lady whom I saw every month of my life.

I used to imagine what Dr. Graham's house looked like – as I did with most people I met, it helped me to work them out. I imagined it to be a beautiful, modern house with many rooms in which the children were not allowed and a number of objects that they were not allowed to touch. I imagined Dr. Graham sitting in her state-of-the-art lounge after a long day at the hospital, sipping wine with her husband and discussing books while listening to classical music.

I started seeing Dr. Graham at Northwick Park Hospital, where I also went for my rheumatology appointments. I remember the department and the room in which I was seen very clearly. We would sit on the chairs outside the room until I was called into Dr. Graham's small, dark room.

My eye was tested on a device called a slit-lamp machine. I would have to sit very still and rest my chin on the chin rest with my forehead pressed against the head rest. There were little pieces of paper towel attached to the chin rest that were torn off and disposed of after each patient. If I didn't see Dr. Graham take them off herself, I would always take one off before putting my chin down. (The cleanliness-induced OCD began in my extremely formative years.)

Once my face was in place, Dr. Graham would sit on the other side looking through what looked like a microscope into my eye. I was always told to look straight ahead at her ear and, as the years passed, I learned to go for long periods of time without blinking to make it easier for the doctors, and to speed up the process for me. As she moved the machine around, the light would reflect off the mirror that was used to see into my eye and it would produce a myriad of beautiful colours. A rainbow. Some sort of promise that things would get better?

Sometimes the light would shine too brightly into my eye, causing me to flinch. Dr. Graham would then take out a miniature magnifying glass to help her see the back of my eye, which apparently was always healthy. Then, the worst part, which I would know was coming when the blue light in the machine came on. I would have to keep very still while Dr. Graham held my eye lids open as she gently poked something into my eye that touched the eyeball itself to test the pressure. For a long time, my pressure was normal, which was a very good thing as it meant I wasn't at risk of glaucoma. This whole process was repeated on my 'good' eye to make sure that that was healthy and, thank goodness, it always was.

I often heard words like 'inflammation' and 'cells'. If there were a lot of cells, this meant that I was having a flare- up, something that happened a few times a year. Mum and I came up with words that made it easy for me to explain how my eye was feeling. It very rarely hurt, but was either 'misty' or 'blurry'. I learned to live with the two, which is why it was hard for my parents to know if something was wrong. Uveitis, except in extreme cases, cannot be seen from the outside, which is why it can be dangerous. Therefore, it was important for me to keep the monthly appointments that monitored the inflammation and cells. Sometimes, if my eye was looking healthy, we were allowed to come back after six weeks or, if we were really lucky, after two months.

For the first few years, Mum would put my eye drops in for me. They had to be kept in the medical room at nursery and school and the medical lady, whom we called Auntie Julie, would administer them for me. I learned to do it myself when I was about eight or nine.

For some reason, I never worried about the condition in my eye, as I always saw the arthritis as being more prominent. It makes more sense now because, at the time, I could feel actual pain and discomfort in my joints, but my eye didn't bother me that much. My parents always seemed so worried about my eye and I just never understood why, until many years later when it started to become a problem.

Chapter 2

Arthritis and the Early years

When I was quite young, the arthritis only affected four joints – my knees and ankles. Childhood pictures show my knees appearing to be very swollen, but this was not always a problem unless I was having a flare. 'Flare' is the term used to describe the increase in symptoms in people with arthritis. Such episodes usually meant that my joints would be more swollen, painful and stiff and I would get very tired.

There are many parts of my childhood throughout which I do not necessarily remember being in pain, but the JRA somehow integrated itself into my whole life. This was something that I worked very hard to fight as I became older.

There are things that seem insignificant now but which must have had an effect on the way I interpreted life. My first memory of being slightly different was when I was in assembly at Nursery. One of the other children – whose face I can still remember so clearly – was sitting on the floor (as we all had to) with his legs in the W position. I was captivated by this and couldn't understand why he could sit in this strange position and find it comfortable. He didn't move once.

In Nursery, I was always sitting on a teacher's lap during assembly because, apparently, I cried all the time until a teacher lifted me up. I never said 'I can't sit on the floor because it hurts', so no one really understood why I cried, not even my parents. I was just known as 'the girl that cries all the time'. As with the ballet classes, this revelation only became apparent years later. It was so simple really, so I'm not sure why no one ever managed to put two and two together. She's got arthritis, she must be in pain. Duh!

By the time I moved to school, I was allowed to sit on a chair during assemblies even though other pupils had to sit on the floor. I can't say that I noticed other children being mean about it, although I do remember the occasional comment: 'why should she sit on a chair when we all have to sit on the floor?' Not everyone at the school understood, but I just had to accept this. I also had to wear fluffy boots in the winter, which kept my ankles warm. They were actually quite nice and I remember Sophie – the same Sophie from nursery – telling me how lucky I was that I could wear such pretty boots when she had to wear patent leather shoes. I think I was lucky, not so much about the shoes but because, despite how cruel children can be, I was never really bullied or tormented. My classmates were always told about my condition and so there was a level of understanding between us.

I loved my primary school, which was a two-minute walk from my house in Maytree Close, Edgware. I always thought that the name of my road was very apt – it looked just how it sounded. There were six houses on each side and there was a big green in the middle where we could play. At the time, most of the families living there had young children or teenagers and after school we would always play there, especially on Friday nights after we had had our Friday night dinner (basically the Jewish version of a Sunday Roast). My friend Lee had dinner with us most nights and after dinner we would take our bowls of chocolate mousse outside and play for hours.

Most of our neighbours were friendly but one was

especially nosey. She would look out of her kitchen window every day to see what was going on and then report back to Mum. It didn't serve me too well later on in life when I was seen to be doing things I shouldn't have been doing.

I had an enjoyable childhood, one that I'm sure many children would be envious of. But everyone has their misfortunes, don't they?

We weren't your typical North West London Jewish family, in that, yes, we were middle class in the sense that we owned our home, we went on holidays and we never wanted for anything. But in a particularly affluent community, I suppose we sat at the lower end. My parents weren't particularly well educated after both coming from working class families who needed them to leave school at fifteen and start working, and they worked in what one would describe as normal jobs but you know what? My mum was around, and all the time. She worked as a secretary at the school we attended so she was always there with us and I wouldn't change that for anything. She taught us, played with us, took us on outings and her general presence meant we were never alone, we were always wanted. She started out as a legal secretary and was very talented in many things and could have gone on to have a great career but she put her family first. There were children who went to Center Parcs when we went to Butlins (the Bognor Regis version, of course), there were those who sported top of the range LA Gear trainers, when we had to wear whatever my dad had found in the market, or those who wore Speedway when we wore Fruit of the Loom (good old Fruit of the Loom). There were those who were educated in how to order from a restaurant menu, when we seldom ate outside of the home. But we had our family and a support network, we were smothered with ridiculous amounts of love and we bloody well had amazing home-cooked meals instead of beans on toast every night and the consequences of those financially-dependent circumstances shape a person for the better in later life.

Back to where we lived: in the same road as my school were a number of shops – a greengrocer's, a grocery store that stocked products from Israel and a newsagent. The greengrocer was a lovely, friendly man named Andrew and we would always chat when we went in for fruit and veg. It was pretty much the same with the other shops: most of the shop keepers knew us by name and knew what was going on in our lives and we liked it that way. London does not have too many close-knit communities anymore, so it was always a nice thought to know that we belonged to one, and despite the politics and disadvantages of belonging to a community that had to know the ins and outs of a ducks arse (as Mum would put it), I always felt like I belonged somewhere, that when the evident disparity of the rest of the country had become so poignant and symbolic of a post mass-immigration era, we were still connected with each other. After all – and most secular Jews would agree – it is not so much about the religious aspect, but the sense of community that keeps us all active in our religion. And for someone who has grown up to view religion in a very different way to how I was supposed to view it – or how I was taught to view it – I can still appreciate and respect that aspect.

Speaking of small communities, my primary school was a relatively small Jewish state school called Rosh Pinah. Everyone knew everyone else – the parents all knew each other and so did the pupils. The older children looked after the younger ones and I don't remember any bullying. The teachers were, in the main, more like friends and we were pretty content. Is it because teachers nowadays are the same age as me that I view them so differently? Because when I was at school I remember the teachers being older, more respected members of the community: hair in a bun, glasses hanging off the end of their noses, tissues hanging out their sleeves and smelling like old fashioned soap. I have friends who are teachers now and to be honest, they make me want to consider home-schooling when I have children.

We loved our headmaster, Mr. Leviton and, to this day, I have never heard of a school head teacher who was liked by so many pupils. He knew each and every one of us by name and treated everyone equally, which is a welcome change when it comes to authoritative figures.

I took my ballet classes at Crystal Arts Theatre School, also in Edgware. The School provided ballet classes for young children, as well as classes in tap, modern dance and drama. All the girls in my primary school class took ballet and, as Mum wanted me to lead as normal a life as possible, I did too. Suffice it to say I managed less than a term as the ballet was too tough for my knees and ankles.

Crystal Arts was owned by a very old lady who had an office in what looked like the steeple of the building, which I think used to be a church. She reminded me of the old bank owner from Mary Poppins; that same scary, old-fashioned look, complete with leathery face, stern features, a back hunched over with a predictable dark mahogany-coloured walking stick in hand to accompany the hunchback, and a high-pitched, crackly old-person voice to finish it off. She was always cold and distant and we were all frightened of her. We held the few pounds that it cost us to take the classes in our pink sequined money bags and we often had to hand it straight to her, making sure we ran away hastily as soon as the money had exchanged hands. Later, when I was about seven, I went back to Crystal Arts and took drama classes every Saturday. It turned out that drama was much more appealing to me than dance, but more of that later.

I also went to a local youth group, Brady Maccabi, on a Sunday afternoon once I turned seven. Although many of my fellow classmates also attended Brady, there were also children from other schools and so we were able to socialise with new people. Brady offered a range of activities to choose from and I opted for art and cookery most weeks. It's probably safe to say that I discovered early on in my life that creativity was an outlet, that I could pour my as-yet undiscovered and unexplored emotions into art. I didn't have arthritis in my hands (yet) so these were all activities in which I could partake without experiencing any pain. I enjoyed the cookery classes as much as the art classes. I enjoyed making things. It didn't really matter what it was as long as I'd started off with nothing, and ended up with something to show for myself.

Predictably enough for a mixed gender early '90s group of kids, not many of them took part in cookery. When we first arrived at the centre in the afternoon, we would all sit in the hall together and each youth leader would shout out what group they'd be taking and we would have to put our hand up if that was the one we wanted to participate in. "Dodgeball", one of the leaders would shout, and there it was, the multitude of eager, sticky young hands thrust up into the air being waved about like some sort of '70s-inspired jazz cabaret show, their heads fiercely moving from side to side like those stupid dogs with moving heads that people put on their dashboards, trying to see who was noticing the fact that they were yearning to play dodgeball, predominately because the owners of all the eager, sticky young hands knew that sport was the best way of showing off. It turns out we are conditioned very early on to understand the paradigm of society and the actions that contribute to it. The girls who joined the boys in playing dodgeball were inevitably 'cool' and subsequently retained their title of 'cool' all through secondary school. And then there was me: "Cookery?" And up my little, shy hand went, hoping to God there would be some other loser, someone preferably relatively unloser-ish who would join me in putting their hand up.

I was, I suppose, a paradox of my own self. I was painfully shy but still craved attention all the time. I wanted everything I did to be better than anyone else so that I would get public praise, especially in school. If someone did something better than me, I would get upset, which was pretty much all the time when it came to maths. I was obsequious in nature, without openly trying to seem obsequious. At home it was always, 'look mummy, look what I did', 'look Aba, look what I made', 'look everyone, please tell me how wonderful I am.' The ego of a person destined for a life of creativity is evident from the earliest age. We just want praise. I also think that having an illness that makes you different to everyone else makes you feel inadequate; you therefore need constant praise to reassure you that you're great.

By the time I was five, my second year at Rosh Pinah, Mum was working at the school part-time as a teaching assistant for Year 2 and I had a new sister, Ilana, who had been born a year earlier. Ilana was a cute baby who looked like a boy until she was about four years old. Reminding her of this gave me great pleasure, whenever I had the chance. My parents were forced to dress her in pink all the time to avoid comments on how gorgeous their 'son' was. We were polar opposites in appearance. She had fair hair that, once it eventually started growing (far too late), was a mass of ringlets whereas my hair had been the first thing that had been seen when I escaped from the womb and it proceeded to grow quickly in dark, straight locks. Ilana was from Mum's side of the family, looks wise, and I was all Vaknine. I remember liking her when she was first born and was excited at the prospect of having a new sister – mostly because she'd gone to the trouble of bringing me Beatrix Potter gifts from Heaven – but when she was a year old, I stopped liking her.

One night, Ilana was in bed and I was downstairs watching

TV with my parents. Ilana started crying and my parents ran upstairs. I could hear Mum telling Dad to 'clean it up'. "I'm here all day every day cleaning up shit and all sorts, you can deal with the sick." My parents were upstairs with Ilana for ages and, even though I hadn't even seen her vomit, I have had a phobia about me or anyone around me being sick ever since. I have had hypnotherapy, counselling and homeopathy to try and relieve me of this phobia, but to no avail. My hypnotist came to the conclusion that it was either something that happened in a past life, or I associate vomit with having the attention taken away from me, which would explain why I both stopped liking my sister and started to fear being sick at around the same time. If this is the case, then I must have been even more attention-seeking than I thought, which I now find particularly depressing and actually, down-right pathetic seeing as my illness meant that the attention was always on me.

Aside from the fact that I disliked my sister most of the time and was extremely horrible to her, like I said earlier, our childhood was pretty awesome for a few reasons but the main one was our holidays to Israel. My dad's family (all thousand of them) lived there, so we would spend our summers as barefoot beach-bums. Before Ilana was born, I had already been there four times. Aba had a huge family – two brothers, five sisters and two half-sisters – plus his mother, my Safta, also had many siblings, which meant that Aba had a multitude of cousins. This is most agreeable when you are a child, because there are always people wanting to make a fuss of you and the fact that we lived abroad and they did not get to see us all the time made them spoil us even more. Except for Safta who had decided that with thirty grandchildren, she would most definitely NOT be buying presents.

We would either stay with Safta or Aba's brother, Asher, who had five children. We would have picnics, beach barbeques and big family parties. There were always colossal amounts of people and even more colossal amounts of food. Three of my dad's siblings moved to South Africa with their diamond businesses during the early '80s and they too would be with us all summer.

I have many fond memories from this time but, (and there's always a but!) somehow, arthritis was forever integrated into my life. My cousins were an energetic bunch and we were always together, but their idea of fun was wetting the grass with the hose and sliding across it to the other side.

From a young age I was acutely aware of my physical inadequacies and the limits they afforded me, so I just stood to the side while they catapulted onto the wet grass and for that I would get a bucket of water thrown over me. They walked around everywhere barefoot, which actually I quite liked as it made me feel free, liberated even, but their feet seemed to be made of asbestos; the marbles floors I could manage, the grass even, but walking to the shops on boiling hot, stony pavement? They were like a bunch of little Mowglis.

One very hot, sticky, typical coastal-Israel night, my uncle and aunt threw a party and all the cousins stayed over, mainly because we had all fallen asleep by the time the party was over; there never seemed to be set bed-times like we had back home, they would run around being as loud and energetic as possible until they physically ran out of all energy and conked out. That was their bed time – usually around midnight, even on school nights. There were about twelve of us sleeping on the floor in one room this particular night. I'd fallen asleep just like everyone else but I remember Mum coming in to put eye drops in my eye. An hour later, she must have thought twice about leaving me in the slumbersome mosh pit of cousins and she picked me up, took me into a different room, changed me into my pyjamas and put me into a bed. They were so unrestrained, my cousins, so unrestricted, like hippies or nomads. I wished I was more like them but Mum would worry about me sleeping on the floor with twelve other kids. The next day wouldn't have been easy on my joints if she'd have left me there. In order to retain my flare-free summers I had to sacrifice these little foibles that would have made me become more a part of it all.

My joints always seemed to be much better when we were in Israel. The heat and sea air changed everything. It was as if the moment I got off that plane and breathed in the familiar smell, disease was washed away in the nearby ocean. My parents often thought about relocating us there for that very reason but it never happened, for several reasons. Although their jobs were reasonably 'portable', as in they didn't have huge career aspirations, Mum did not want to leave my grandparents. The doctors advised us that if we did move to Israel, we should move to the south, to the more arid areas but Aba's family lived in the coastal town of Netanya. What would've been the point of moving there to not be near everyone? And although yes, humidity isn't the best thing for arthritis, I was always in better health when I was there. Not everything is black and white when it comes to health.

We did make many visits to the arid area of the Dead Sea and we were lucky that it was so accessible for us. People travel from all over the world with all sorts of illnesses to bathe in the Dead Sea waters and cover their bodies in Dead Sea mud, both of which are said to have healing properties.

I loved going to the Dead Sea. We would usually be accompanied by members of the Vaknine family from Netanya, all jumping into trucks to head down there. The shores of the Dead Sea are the lowest point on the Earth's surface and you can feel the pressure in your ears as the car descends down the winding road to the Dead Sea. Once we got there, it was heaven. Being at the Dead Sea is like being in a different world, an almost mystical, enigmatic place. It is so isolated and far away from reality. I think this is what we all liked about it. Everyone could escape from their lives for a few days.

We stayed in a hotel with sulphur baths, mud treatments and all the other wonderful treats that came part and parcel with being at the Dead Sea. The hotel boasted many different swimming pools. The sulphur baths reeked of eggs, which made me feel sick for a bit. These baths were hot and very relaxing and the sulphur content was supposed to do wonders for healing. Because I couldn't bear the smell, it took a while to get me in there, but eventually Mum was able to make me do my exercises in the water to loosen up my joints.

Later in the day, when the heat had lessened, we would head for the beach, loaded down with food, of course, because God forbid the Vaknines (if at this point in the book you're still wondering how to pronounce Vaknine, its VAKNEEN. It is for Moroccan Israelis what Smith is for Brits) shouldn't eat for a few hours. We put up a small tent for those who wanted some shade and arranged the food and drink on our beach picnic table. Even though we were only a few minutes from the hotel, my family never went anywhere without a picnic table and cooler boxes. The kids would run around and play, the adults would sit on folding chairs eating fruits and nuts and drinking coffee from Thermos's. These are some of the best memories of my life.

The most wonderful thing about the Dead Sea is that people float on top of it. The salt and mineral content is so high that no creatures can live in it, hence the name. You can't drown in the Dead Sea. Some bathers even take plastic chairs into the water and float around reading their newspapers. The main problem with all that salt though, is that if you have an open wound, it really stings, and that's not the only thing that stings; you can't stay in for too long!

The mud baths were also a lot of fun for some, but as I was a child with a hatred of dirt and mess, covering my body in mud did not really appeal but of course, as ever, I had to do it because 'it was good for me'.

I will never forget that depressing feeling one experiences as a child when a holiday comes to an end and things go back to normal. For some reason it's not as bad when you're an adult, maybe because we understand and accept the realities of life, but as a child, coming home from holiday felt like the end of the world.

England was not all bad though, as we had many family outings, trips and holidays. During the Easter / Passover holidays, we would go to Thorpe Park – a huge theme park an hour out of London. We would join up with my friends and their families, but the dads never came with us.

I think men these days are far more hands-on, far more interested in being a part of their childrens' day-to-day lives. When I was young, we would never even question why the dads weren't with us. They worked and that was all there was to it, even on the weekends.

My friend Rachel's mother had a huge foreign car with left-hand drive. It may have been old but was big enough to accommodate me, Mum and Ilana, as well as Rachel and her mother, brother and sister. We didn't spend much time worrying about Health and Safety in those days...

For my eighth birthday, Nanny and Poppa bought me a Walkman, which I would always take on our day trips, and while the other kids were playing eye spy or looking to count how many red cars they saw, I sat bopping my head to Take That and Michael Jackson. I don't think there's any part of my life where there isn't a song or artist whose music I don't associate with it. Music was – and still is – everything for me.

Once we got to Thorpe Park, we would all meet up and the first thing we would do, of course, was eat. I was jealous –

always jealous of something – that my best friend Simi (my best friend to this day) was wearing a pretty dress when I had to wear a thick tracksuit. When I said earlier that despite my wonderful childhood, JRA always somehow integrated itself into my life, this is why. There was always something reminding me that I couldn't be the same as everyone else. "You can't wear a dress to a theme park because you need to have your knees protected," Mum would say. Bless her. She thought of everything she could to keep me safe.

By the time the day was over and we piled in the car to go home, we were all exhausted and slept the whole way back. But I would moan about the tracksuit *vs* dress situation for days, if not weeks. I had a knack of not being able to let things go. Much to my detriment, I still do.

Mum spent pretty much all her time with us and it's only now as I've gotten older and my friends are starting to have children that I realise how lucky we were to have a mum that was always around. Aside from our day trips during the holidays, she'd take us to see the latest Disney movie at our local cinema on a Saturday or Sunday afternoon – a real treat, especially as we were allowed popcorn or ice cream.

In the summer we went for day trips to Westcliff-on-Sea with Nanny and Poppa. We would play on the murky, grainy English beaches and, while spooning the pebbly detritus into my red plastic bucket, I would wonder why we had to have stony beaches when Israel had sandy ones. These memories sit with me in such a beautiful way. I remember being happy, content, excited about life, unperturbed by my looming disability while we ended our day with fish and chips in one of the seaside restaurants holding onto the little colourful windmills that Nanny and Poppa had bought us.

Nanny and Poppa were constant fixtures in our lives and I treasure the memories of simple days with them; days when I was ill and off school and would spend the day at their house playing Uno with Nanny or watching Countdown under a blanket with Poppa while Nanny made dinner in the kitchen. Boiled potatoes and rose water; that's what their house always smelled like. God I miss it. I miss my Nanny's gentle, unselfish kindness and Poppa's grandfatherly love.

Boiled potatoes may have been the way forward at Nanny's who, bless her, wasn't much of a cook, but Fridays at home were sensational. Mum learned Moroccan cooking from Safta and boy was she good at it. She would spend the whole day on Friday cooking and cleaning while Ilana and I would have to occupy ourselves, playing or fighting over the remote control in the lounge. The nostalgic smell still permeates through my nostrils to this day and fills me with smiles. Coriander, chillies, roast chicken, cakes, a spicy Moroccan tomato sauce called *matbucha* bubbling on the stove, artichokes steaming in a large saucepan next to it and some sort of soup heating away nearby. A culmination of culinary wonders mixed in with cleaning products. It still smells like that at Mum's house on a Friday and I'll never grow tired of it.

Ilana and I were always encouraged musically. In the Jewish community of North West London, most parents opt to provide their children with childhood piano or violin lessons in the hope that their child will hold some talent, but they almost always hope that the child doesn't want to take up music professionally. Musicians are always out of work, don't you know. By secondary school the lesson taught is the idea that it is great to have a talent and to show it off, but the 'wonders' of law and the banal art of filing a tax return are really the things that matter. I find most Jews to be grafters, brought up to know that they have to work hard and make a good living and make something of themselves because if they don't, no one will give it to them, we don't take handouts. This can only be a good thing for them and for society and I'm proud to come from a community with a strong work ethic but creativity was never shunned in our family; we were always a little bit different. Mum was a great singer herself and was a member of a choir, and was always highly creative. She always wanted us to play musical instruments. When I was seven years old (it seems to me through writing this that lots of things took place when I was seven), Mum decided it was about time that I started learning. She asked me which instrument I'd like to learn. I thought about the harp, strangely, but decided I was already too different to everyone else to choose a medieval instrument of gargantuan proportions (there was a boy in school who played the tuba and it was bigger than him and we all laughed at him), so I settled on the guitar. Mum's choir director was a music teacher and I started going to him for lessons once a week. I didn't just enjoy playing the guitar, I was really good at it and of course it meant I could perform to family and friends and get praise which, let's be honest, was my favourite part.

I was studying classical guitar, which was quite difficult but I suppose easier to learn the younger you are, and I picked it up fairly quickly. My teacher asked me to join him and some of the older students in a recital one Sunday afternoon. I don't remember much about it, but I do remember being backstage practicing all day. We played so much that we were given special cream to rub into our fingers where the guitar strings would have made a dent. We performed on stage in front of quite a large audience and I don't remember being nervous at all. I began to take guitar examinations and started taking part in school assemblies too, alongside Dalia, the only other girl in the school who played guitar. We played classical songs, like Greensleeves and some Mozart pieces, and looking back now, that's not bad for the seven year old who couldn't play dodgeball. It was something I could do that others couldn't, and I was always looking for more of these things. Like the more I could do that others couldn't, the more it would validate me and balance out my inadequacies in other areas.

Ilana started roller-blading which looked slightly appealing but a little too dangerous for me, but I was jealous of the fact that she had no limitations and no fear of getting hurt. I wasn't ready for roller-blades so I asked Mum to buy me a skateboard. She did, of course, doing anything she could to make me feel more normal but I was never able to bring myself to actually stand on it. I just sat straddling it pushing myself along while Ilana sped past on her blades.

Music was another member of our family. One of my friends used to say that being in my house was like being in a musical, as we would suddenly burst into song at any given moment. And it was true; whenever someone said something that resembled a line from a song, we would all start singing. Ilana had a great voice and started taking singing lessons. We thought there was a possibility she could be a mini Charlotte Church at one point, but she never followed it through.

Due to our parents' diverse music collection, Ilana and I grew up listening to a much more eclectic mix of music than just the songs we heard on Disney films. Aba preferred old French and Italian music, the likes of Edith Piaf, Franco Zerilli and Enrico Macias, as well as Arab-Andalusian music from Morocco, Israel and Spain (think Gypsy Kings meets Arabian nights). A cacophony of popular Moroccan songs that I knew all the words to but had no idea what they meant, was always the soundtrack to parties at our house. Nanny and Poppa, even with fifty years filling the hole between the war and the '90s, never tired of playing the old war songs by Dame Vera Lynn, Flanagan and Allen and Glenn Miller, and Mum brought us up on the Beatles, '50s Rock and Roll, Simon and Garfunkel and Motown, and later on came The Divas: Celine Dion, Barbara Streisand, Shirley Bassey, Bette Midler, Mariah Carey and Whitney Houston. Ilana and I would drown ourselves in an ensemble of our best costume jewellery, silk scarves and

Mum's heels and stand at the top of the stairs crooning 'Goldfinger' and 'The Power of Love' at the top of our tiny, strained voices like wailing banshees. Our favourite cassette tape was a compilation of love songs from the '50s like Teenager in Love, Only You and Those Magic Changes – this was a real winner with us.

After Nanny and Poppa bought me my first Walkman, I asked Mum to take me to Loppylugs – a record shop and absolute institution in Edgware that, had I have been old enough, I would have campaigned to keep open. I even remember what it smelled like in there; the smell of new records, aftershave and the faint, stale smell of cigarettes. On my first trip to Loppylugs I made two purchases – the first two albums I ever bought: Michael Jackson's Bad and Jason Donovan's Greatest Hits. Jason Donovan was the first male I ever really displayed sexual feelings for. Well, not sexual, I was too young, but feelings that were not purely platonic. He was my first celebrity crush. And there were many to follow.

Somewhere within the mishmash of all that eclecticism, Hip Hop weaseled its way in. I started taking a liking to rappers like Tupac, Biggie and Snoop Doggy Dogg. This led into a love of gangster movies and books. Strange, you might think, for a nine year-old Jewish girl from North West London to be watching The Godfather and Scarface and listening to songs about rappers and their turf wars. It really was strange, I don't even know how I came across it – MTV maybe? Out of all the music I had heard growing up, and there was lots of it, Gangster Rap was never something played in our house, funnily enough. It just slithered its way into my life somehow.

Through Hip Hop and MTV, I came across classic R&B and Soul and, from a very young age, this music played a huge part in my life. My Walkman went with me everywhere and, with the help of Loppylugs, I gradually moved away from New Kids on the Block and Jason Donovan to Mary J. Blige, Salt 'n' Pepa,

Jodeci, En Vogue, Color Me Bad and Boyz II Men.

When I look back, no matter what happened with my health, I am lucky enough to be able to say that I have great memories from my childhood, memories that although perhaps tainted here and there with pain, ones that will nevertheless stay with me forever and be held close as some of the best of my life.

Chapter 3

Hospitals and Homeopaths

When I was first diagnosed with arthritis, the doctors didn't have many options. Most children with arthritis were given daily oral steroids, but taking steroids for long periods of time can cause many side effects. Long-term side effects include osteoporosis, weight gain, muscle damage and increased risk of infection – along with a bunch of other ones that aren't listed on the packet. None of these were risks my parents were prepared to take with a two-year old with her whole life ahead of her, so they decided against the steroids. At the time, this was more or less the only medication available for people with arthritis.

Aba worked as a market trader selling children's clothes. At the time, the markets were booming so 'market trader' wasn't as frowned upon as belonging to the lower echelons of society as it is today. He earned a good enough wage and I benefitted greatly from the fact that he sold children's clothes. At the time that my parents were discussing how to relieve the swelling in my joints, Aba found that his stall one day was opposite a man with a book stall. He had worked in that market for years and had never seen a bookseller near him before.

On that particular day, there was a red book on the stall

that Aba always said 'jumped out' at him. He walked over and picked up the book and, although we cannot remember the exact title, it was to do with how to treat arthritis alternatively. Mum had wanted to take the alternative route but had not been sure where to start and, when Aba bought this book home, it made up her mind.

This really changed the course of my life. I genuinely believe that if we had not followed alternative therapies, my life would be very different now. The book explained about the importance of diet and gave an insight into homeopathy and how it worked. Mum found out about the Royal London Homeopathic Hospital in Great Ormond Street. It was available on the NHS which was reassuring as homeopathy was extremely expensive but when Mum approached our GP to get a referral, she was told that there was a five-year waiting list. We could not wait that long, so Mum investigated other homeopathic options, in spite of being advised against this route by many doctors at the hospital: "Don't waste your money, Mrs. Vaknine, there's no proof that any of that stuff works." Alternative therapies were approached with great trepidation in those days (still are really), but Mum was adamant that it would be better for me than the steroids. I mean really, if there is an option to treat naturally instead of pumping your two year old full of chemicals, why wouldn't you try it as a first resort instead of last? Pharmaceutical companies. Bureaucracy. Money. More of that later.

After some research and more time in the library, she found a homeopathic dietician in Harley Street, an elderly gentleman who was very pleased that we had decided to take this route. He explained that, with a potentially long-term illness such as this, it would be best to avoid the steroids because of the side effects. After the feeling of guilt, like it is their fault that this has happened to their child, most parents then go into a state of denial. They believe that this illness cannot possibly be here for the rest of their lives and it will go away, so the best thing to do is to take all the medications the doctors are offering and hope that this helps get rid of it as quickly as possible. The problem with that is that if the illness doesn't go away, which in most cases it doesn't, (and that sentence might not appeal to you but it doesn't. Better to know early on), the child becomes accustomed to the medications and of course all of the medications come with side effects. So looking for alternative options was very brave of my parents and I can only thank the powers that be for making them feel there were other options.

Just in case you were wondering, after the guilt and denial comes fear. The fear that actually this illness might be here for the rest of her life and there is absolutely nothing you can do to stop it.

We only saw this dietician twice, but he gave me a strict diet to which I had to adhere. I was no longer allowed wheat, gluten, dairy, acidic foods such as pickles or oranges and anything that came in aluminium cartons, such as fruit juices. This was particularly tough on Mum as she was expected to explain to a two-year old that she could not eat what her friends were having. For some reason, though, just before my second birthday, I had completely gone off milk and all dairy products. The dietician said that this was my body's way of telling me that it wasn't good for me (not that diary is good for us anyway. Again, more of that later). Children often have this kind of sixth sense, so if the body tells them something isn't good for them, they don't eat it, rather like when children are full, they will stop eating because their bodies tell them they've had enough. Adults, on the other hand, do not know how to listen to their bodies. If something is bad for them, they will still eat it if they want it and, even if they are full, they will carry on eating if they want to.

Oddly enough, I didn't really like food at all when I was young. Mum says I lived on 'air pies' from the ages of two to six. All I ever wanted was apple juice and I drank gallons of it every day. Maybe there is something in apples that my body needed and craved.

Mum would ask the doctors why I didn't eat and she worried dreadfully about it. There really is nothing worse for a mother than a child that will not eat, and for a Jewish mother with a sick child, well, this was the worst thing possible, especially coming from our Israeli background where everything – and I mean everything – revolves around food. If people were invited over, it was to eat. Even if they were only coming for 'coffee', this meant home-made cakes, biscuits and probably some sort of meal later on. The doctor whom Mum spoke to about this – who happened to be a Jewish doctor from South Africa – told her that "if a child is hungry, she will eat, especially a Jewish child. So don't worry too much."

We continued with my diet and, when I was four, we found The Homeopathic Centre in Edgware High Street and its location couldn't have been more convenient. We were met by Ian, a very friendly, welcoming man, who explained to us how it all worked and that there was a herbalist, Beatrice, whom we could see if we wished. We made an appointment to see her and, although I didn't really enjoy going as it seemed a chore for me, it came as a welcome distraction from the hospitals. I didn't ever understand why I went nearly once a week to see Beatrice, but it wasn't un-enjoyable. I did, however, hate the appointment room, which was small, dark and dismal and reminded me of nightmares, especially in the winter when we went after school and it was dark already. The window in the room was tiny and had bars across it, like in a prison, and you could see the alleyway at the back of the shop. I never liked the smell of the homeopathic herbs and remedies.

My appointments would last usually about an hour and then, depending on what had been said, my remedy would be selected. The remedies usually came in dissolving tablet form but sometimes as drops that I would put under my tongue. They tasted kind of bland but a little bit like alcohol. As Mum had been giving me a tonic called Kindervital, a brown liquid that tasted absolutely putrid, I had become accustomed to strange tastes. Mum also made me drink nettle juice and nettle tea as often as I would take it.

Most of the talking in these sessions went on between Beatrice and Mum. Before Beatrice talked to me, she would give me a piece of paper and some crayons and ask me to draw a picture. Every time, I would hit the crayons onto the paper to make large dots and do that, with force, all over the paper. Beatrice would later evaluate this behaviour, but I am not sure what the final verdict was. She did try and talk to me too. She always asked me about my dreams. The subconscious carries a lot of information that our conscious minds do not know about, or cannot see, but which comes out through dreams. This is why most dreams can be interpreted into something that is relevant in our lives. I used to dream a lot about houses. In fact, most weeks I would have at least one dream about houses, or one house in particular. The dreams would feature all sorts of houses; big ones, small ones, nicely decorated ones, scary ones, secret passageways (these were my favourite), houses with farms and big gardens and houses in which, no matter how long you walked through them, you never quite came to the end.

I have heard different interpretations over the years for what these dreams meant. One reason could be that, as dreaming of a house usually refers to various aspects of the self, never being able to find the end of the house could have been never knowing when things in my life would come to an end, and dreaming of secret passageways and rooms into which I could not go signified the lack of control that I had in my life, not being able to do what I really wanted. Some people may argue that all this is too deep for a four-year old mind to conjure up and they may be right, but I believe that the soul has no age and therefore the subconscious mind is more powerful than we understand.

A more believable answer for why I dreamed of houses so much could be that I grew up to be an interior designer, perhaps I was seeing a part of my future... I guess we'll never know.

Beatrice would always say that I had lovely red lips, which made me look as if I was wearing lipstick. She said it was unusual for a child with chronic pain to have any colour in their lips and so I enjoyed this thought. I did, however, have very dark, black/purple circles under my eyes all the time, which I hated with a passion and I tried everything I could to cover them up. My friend Lee and I raided her mother's toiletries cupboard once, put a big blob of white cream under my eyes and then stuck talcum powder on top, hoping that this might stain the skin under my eyes white. Only later on in life would I learn about the wonderful gift of make-up. The bags under my eyes were caused by pain and, after a few years of experiencing this pain, they never went away. Looking at my face in the mirror without concealer is a constant reminder of that pain.

At the same time that I was seeing Beatrice, I was transferred to another rheumatologist. Dr. Ansell was leaving full time practice to spend more time on research, so she handed her clinic over to Dr. Smith, later to become Professor Smith.

Dr. Smith was one of the best in her field, but I never felt a connection with her. She always carried out a thorough check-up, telling me to take off my shoes, socks and trousers or skirt and making me walk from one side of the room to the other just wearing my knickers. She would then ask me to pick things up with my toes, stand on tiptoes and then back onto my heels, and then check the movement of my joints while I lay on her examination bed. She would measure my legs by placing the tape measure on my hips, but I was so ticklish that I would laugh and squirm and she could never get the tape measure in the right place, which aggravated her greatly. Mum explained to Dr. Smith that I never complained, even when the joints seemed inflamed. Dr. Smith replied that children get used to something and think it is normal, therefore they do not complain because they know no different. My joints were very hyper-mobile (known then as double-jointed), which is why, when I was young, I had no problem with my mobility and Dr. Smith was able to move my legs in any way she wanted. A misconception made by many less experienced rheumatologists is that because the joints have great mobility, there must be no swelling. They forget that most JRA kids are hyper-mobile and therefore the mobility is always exaggerated despite present swelling.

I was able to do things with my hands that I thought everyone could do until, one day, someone at school said that what I did with my thumb was disgusting. I went around the playground asking everyone if they could do it and no one else could. I was amazed and thought it was pretty cool that I had a little party trick that no one else could do. At this time I didn't have arthritis in my hands, but my fingers and thumbs could literally move any way I bent them so, from a very young age, I clicked my fingers a lot and found it funny when people would say 'be careful, if you keep doing that you'll get arthritis'.

Dr. Smith enrolled me into weekly group physiotherapy sessions with other children who had arthritis. I enjoyed these groups a lot. I think this was mainly because it gave me the opportunity to be with a group of children who were going through the same as me and, although as children we never spoke about it to each other, and although people might have expected us to hate being at the hospital, we all felt at ease in that hospital gym. I was the youngest apart from one other girl who was just two years old, the same age I was when I was diagnosed. There was also a girl with Down's Syndrome and some other girls, but only one boy. We sat in a circle and the physiotherapist would make us all do the same exercises with our legs. It was comforting to know that they were all in some sort of pain, unlike in school where PE classes meant that I would be in pain but everyone else would be having a great time. I also attended group hydrotherapy sessions.

The main thing is that I enjoyed and looked forward to my weekly sessions of physio and hydro and not just because it meant I could leave school early. Children's hydro sessions involve two or three physiotherapists being in the pool too and parents standing around the pool wearing awful blue plastic overshoes. It was comforting to know that Mum was there watching me and I would show off, as usual, so she could see that I was doing well. Much of the time I had much better movement than most of the other children. I was the only one who was not taking steroids, so I was not slowed down by fatigue and didn't have the problem of my bones being affected by the drugs. Unless I was going through a flare-up, I was generally energetic and playful and so there was a visible difference between the others and me.

When I say energetic, I mean in comparison with other children with arthritis. Next to my own friends, I seemed quite different. When my friends had sleepovers, I rarely joined in. I got tired so early that I was just happy to be put to bed by 7.00pm and I knew that if I slept at a friend's house, I would be up a lot later. I never understood why my friends fought their parents to stay up later and, why it was such a treat. For me, the treat was to be in bed.

As I became older, my friends would tease me about going to bed so early. According to them, I should have at least stayed up late enough to watch Eastenders at 7:30. I never realised at the time why I was the only one who didn't like staying up late, but even twenty years down the line I still had the same problem and so it makes sense. Pain drains energy from you. When all your energy is being used up being in and fighting pain, you have no energy left for anything else. By the end of the day, all you want to do is sleep. Pain can do a lot of things to you, but one thing that many people who don't suffer with chronic pain cannot understand is just how tiring it is. Arthritis, being an auto-immune disease, also drains energy, because the immune system is constantly working overtime. Once I grew up and realised there were reasons for these strange behavioural patterns of mine that were so different to all of my friends, it made it much easier to accept and know that no one could make fun of that any more.

I have always felt the cold. My hands and feet are always cold and I have to wear several layers of clothing, so going into a hot hydro pool was bliss to start with, but not for long. After a while, the room became so hot that I could feel the condensation dripping down the windows all over my body. There was a huge picture of dolphins in the sea on the wall behind the pool and I used to imagine myself jumping out of this hot, sweaty pool into the cool, crisp sea to join the beautiful dolphins. Years later, I did get to swim with dolphins and the significance wasn't lost.

I also enjoyed showing off my swimming skills in the hydro pool. Ever since my diagnosis, Mum had taken me to swimming lessons every Saturday, as the doctors had said that swimming is great to loosen the joints and aid mobility. As you can probably tell by now, my mum did everything humanly possible to keep me as normal and mobile as possible and keep the arthritis at bay. Were it not for all her efforts when I was young, my childhood would have been very different.

I always looked forward to swimming lessons. We would head down to Borehamwood swimming pool, a huge pool with three diving boards; one close to the water, one half-way up and one so high that I only once had the courage to jump off and I jumped and didn't dive, so I hated it. Every few months, we would have swimming tests for each level and, if I passed, I received a badge made of fabric that Mum would sew onto my swimming costume. I loved that costume and still have all the badges. I always felt that swimming was the one thing I could do that I was better at doing than all the children at school. They could all run, dance, play football (and dodgeball) and sit cross-legged comfortably but, in the pool, I was the best.

So I had a swimming party for my sixth birthday. What a great idea, I thought, especially when some of the children said that they couldn't swim. I was selfishly happy – I loved the fact that there was something that I could do better. Mum and Aba hired out the whole venue for the day. There was a huge inflatable octopus in the centre of the pool and the children who were not strong swimmers could stay in the shallow end. Mum was in the pool helping all those children whose parents had not come and I took advantage of the chance to show off. I swam to the deep end, did back flips, somersaults and handstands in the water and took some of my friends to the lower diving board.

At the party lunch, Mum and Nanny presented me with an amazing cake in the shape of a mini swimming pool with miniature people jumping into it. It was the best birthday anyone could have asked for and all the guests agreed that it was the most fun they had had at a birthday party.

The following year, for my seventh birthday, I had a pizza party at a restaurant where we all made our own pizzas. It was great fun and another way for me to enjoy myself without being in pain.

The homeopathy was helping my body to fight the arthritis without putting any chemicals in my body and, aside from the odd cold and throat infection, I was generally healthy.

On a beautiful spring day in June 1991, I was sitting in Miss. Sommerfeld's year 2 class at school learning about John Major and Michael Heseltine (how strange that I remember this), when my eye started feeling strange. I told my teacher that I had to get my sunglasses out of my bag that sat on my peg just outside the classroom, but I was not allowed. I suppose she thought that everyone in the class was being affected by the sun coming through the window and that I sounded like a bit of a princess, but I knew that something was wrong and that my parents had bought the sunglasses to stop my eyes being exposed to too much sun. Because I wasn't allowed to go, I shut my mouth and sat in silence until the end of class. When school finished I went into the playground and the look on Mum's face was one that I had never seen before and don't think I've seen since. She put me into the car and rushed me to A&E, from where I was sent to St. Thomas' Hospital. I loved St. Thomas' because it was on the River Thames and right next to Big Ben. My eye had turned a strange shade of grey and the cells that Dr. Graham had talked about had become visible to the human eye, which was very rare.

I was having a severe flare-up of the uveitis. I was sent up to Rainbow Ward. I didn't really understand what was going on, but I was quite comfortable in hospital. It is strange when I think about it now, how much I liked being in hospital. Most kids who grow up with hospitals as their second home despise the places, but I felt at home. It didn't bother me.

The doctors kept me very calm as they sat me down and asked me some questions to make sure I understood what was going on. They were going to put me to sleep the next morning and inject steroid into my eye to reduce the inflammation that was causing my eye to be so misty that it looked like there was a constant white cloud in front of it.

Mum stayed with me in the ward that night. There was a

baby there whose parents were not with him and this upset Mum, which in turn upset me. How could any mother who is offered a bed and the opportunity to stay with her one year old baby refuse?

That night, I was down as 'nil by mouth' and was missing my apple juice but, eventually, I fell asleep. The next morning I was taken down to the operating theatre.

I don't really remember being scared, but Mum was holding my hand while a big, ugly, smelly, rubber mask was put over my face and this made me fall asleep. I cannot tell you exactly what I dreamed about, but I do remember that I had nightmares about monsters and ghosts and anything else frightening and I made Mum promise not to let them give me that gas again. Next time, I would be brave and have the injection to put me to sleep.

I woke up in recovery with a patch over my eye and, for some reason, when the nurse asked if I wanted anything, the first thing I asked for was Five Alive, but all they brought me was water, so I didn't see the point in them asking me what I wanted. I was taken back up to the ward, where Aba, Nanny and Poppa were waiting for me. I am not exactly sure where poor Ilana was throughout all of this.

I stayed in for about five days so that they could monitor me, as the flare-up had been so sudden and acute that they had to observe it carefully. A few days after my operation, Mum took me to the pay phones and I called my best friend, Simi. She was the only person I wanted to call. All the children in my class at school had made me a beautiful card and Simi brought it to the hospital for me. It was very big and everyone had written something. A few days after I left hospital, during the Friday afternoon assembly that we had every week to wish everyone a good Sabbath, Mum took me into school to say thank you. Although my eye was closed, which must have looked a bit strange, I liked the fact that I walked into school in dungarees when everyone else was in uniform.

I was asked a lot of questions by everyone and enjoyed all the attention, but after about half an hour Mum said it was too much for me and took me home. Although I had had one other steroid injection in my eye before this incident, this was the first of many that I remember and not all of them held such nice memories.

My eye stayed shut for a few months, which looked really strange. It opened eventually, but never really looked the same after that injection. Once I was back at school, my routine went back to normal.

Sports Day was always an event that I dreaded. Apart from the egg and spoon race, everything else required speed, which was something I did not have. I gave it a go all the same. The only reason I did enjoy Sports Day was because parents of students were allowed to bring their dogs with. I always loved animals and, between the ages of seven and fourteen, I was sure that I was going to be a vet when I grew up. It was only when I realised that I had to study maths at A-level I decided against it. I was always so bad with numbers that I was sure I had some sort of 'number dyslexia'. It got worse as I got older – quite the opposite of what I expected.

When I was three, on the way home from nursery, Aba told me that there was a surprise for me at home and, when I got there, there was a German Shepherd puppy waiting in the kitchen. She was about to be put down because no one wanted her and so Aba decided to rescue her. I named her Scruffy after a dog in one of my favourite cartoons and she was beautiful. I will never forget how elated I was when I saw her and was told she was mine. I loved playing with her, coming home to see her after nursery and taking her to the park. I felt a deep bond towards animals and loved them, all of them. I wanted to be around them all the time. Scruffy grew and grew and grew until she was bigger than me and eating everything from furniture to shoes. My parents had done a good thing adopting her but they didn't have the time to devote to a dog, especially such a demanding breed. They both worked full time and really that's just selfish. They couldn't devote the time to train her properly and because of that she became a nuisance – well, not to me.

After less than a year of owning Scruffy, Mum became pregnant with Ilana and that was the final straw for them. They were both out at work every day, expecting another child and had another child with health problems to look after. We gave Scruffy to a lady who had other dogs and lived on a farm – or so I was told. It was a nice thought and at the time I was happy because she was being looked after and was in a better place, where she could have more room to run around, but I missed her dreadfully. After that I pestered my parents for another dog all the time, but they never gave in, and Sports Day was the one day that I could play with everyone else's dogs.

Luckily, it was usually sunny on Sports Day. We used the grounds of Broadfields Primary School, which was round the corner from Rosh Pinah, because we didn't have enough room for such an event. We would walk there holding hands with our buddy - mine always being my Rachel or Simi and when we arrived we would sit in our designated areas, waiting for the games to start. Most of the parents would be there to watch us. Aba never usually came because he was working, but Mum was always there and always participated in the Mothers' Race - she even won once. I would get butterflies in my stomach as the time for the first race approached, feeling sick with nerves knowing that everyone would be seeing how dreadful I was at running. I wondered if they would see that I ran abnormally and whether or not they noticed my swollen knees. I hoped onlookers were not aware of my differences, but was always self-conscious enough to be overtaken with the worry that they were. I would watch Nicole - the sportiest girl in our class - win every race, every year. So, I always tried to stay as far away from her as I could, so no one would notice how far behind her I was.

One year, I remember having significantly more difficulty with the races and so I spent most of that day speaking to Gary Brown. Gary was a boy in the year above me who was born without a voice box and was the only other person in the school (that I was aware of) who had a physical disability. He had a helper with him during school hours, whose name was Joan. I remember her so well. Being in a Jewish School, she was probably the first black lady I had ever seen (how sheltered we were). Joan would always ask if I was OK and would help me in any way she could.

Gary had to carry around a box with different pieces of equipment to help him breathe and talk. He and I spent that whole day talking to each other between races, helping each other reach the end of the next one, giving each other motivation. At the time I don't think we realised that is what we were doing, as we were too young, but we helped each other all the same and both our mothers were in tears as they watched. Gary and I didn't understand why they cried so much – now, of course, I can see why.

Around the same time, I was sent to the podiatry clinic in Northwick Park to get fitted for insoles for my shoes. These had three functions. Firstly, the arthritis had affected the way that my legs had grown and one was now longer than the other, so the insole in one of the shoes was lower than the other one. Secondly, in order to ease the pain, I would walk in all sorts of strange ways, sometimes with my feet facing inwards, and at other times with my ankles bending inwards or even on the sides of my feet. After about six years, this had affected my feet. Thirdly, they were there as another reminder of how different I was.

One would have thought that I would have resented all the hospital appointments, but, like I said earlier, I didn't – I enjoyed the fact that I could leave school early, or go in late, depending on when the appointment was. Mum said that I was never really a high-flier at school, which I now resent. I don't think the school systems are set up in a way to push children to find their potential. Mum was right in a way, I was middle of the road, but there was a thirst for knowledge and a blob of intelligence in there somewhere. The really clever kids are pushed because they have potential, and the ones with special needs are helped loads more for obvious reasons, but us middle-of-the-road kids have no chance in a state school. No one was going to delve deep enough to find my as yet unknown passions. Like I said, school systems are not set up like this and they have become one of a number of establishments that I have an increasing problem with for that very reason. Plus, I hated hearing Mum talk about me in any way that wasn't utterly positive. She was not trying to put me down, quite the opposite in fact, as she always encouraged me in everything I wanted to do. She just made assumptions on how I was doing academically and forewarned me before I was old enough to decide for myself. I tried hard at the subjects I enjoyed, such as history and science, failed miserably at maths, and excelled only in art, Hebrew and, occasionally, English.

I was never the most confident of children so I suppose I underestimated my academic abilities and decided from a young age that I was 'average'. I was not the most clever person around, but I was certainly not the most stupid but I succumbed to 'average' early on. This was what I always heard teachers and parents saying; 'she's not a highflyer, but she'll do OK, she's average.' I suppose if you hear something enough you believe it. It turns out they were wrong but it took near on two decades for me to figure this out and I had to do it on my own, to wonder why I was so inquisitive, why I had a thirst for knowledge and read history books and plays and philosophy and knew information on subjects that most of my peers had never heard about. You don't need to be getting As in maths to be clever. Another type of 'bright' comes from those who are hungry for knowledge. I find now that those people are usually the most intelligent because they *want* to learn, they are not forced into it. I had the abilities, they were always there but no one saw it in me at a young age.

I suppose my parents and teachers could have seen what sort of child I was by my intensity, but they just saw it as a flaw, an annoyance. Aside from being a perfectionist and getting frustrated at school work if I didn't understand it from the very beginning, I was intense a lot of the time; filled with emotions and acutely aware of the emotions of others.

Like everything else, when you are a child you don't realise what is commonplace and what is different or strange but thinking about it now, my awareness and absorption of other people's emotions was not normal for a young child. From as early as I can remember – and my memories go back as far as around two years old – I remember sort of 'feeling' what others were feeling. When I was about six, my mum had found out that a friend of hers had died and she didn't want to cry in front of me. She took herself to the bath after the brother of this friend had called to tell her but I had this overwhelming sensation of melancholy within me and I knew it was coming from Mum. Nowadays I'd call it an aura, you can, after all, feel people's energies when they emit them, it's just that some people are more open to acknowledging or recognising it and even then as a very young child, I was so open to other people's emotions. I absorbed them as if they were my own and felt what they were feeling. I gently knocked on the bathroom door and asked Mum if I could come in. She said yes and tried to dry away her tears but I said, "What's wrong

Mummy? Why are you sad?" "A friend of mine died today, you remember the lady who lives round the corner? She's gone to heaven so I'm a bit sad that I won't see her anymore," Mum said. "I'm sorry you're sad Mummy. I'm sad too."

At the time I don't suppose Mum understood why I was sad, or she may have thought I was sad *for* her, or sad because I was in pain. What she didn't realise was that because she was sad I was sad, I felt what she was feeling.

Another time I remember was when Nanny came to pick me up from school and I got a shock to see her waiting for me in the playground instead of Mum. She told me that Mummy was at home because she wasn't well. Now, I've looked after many children over the years and I can honestly say that at that age (six), children aren't really fussed. They know Mummy will get better and that's that. When Nanny told me Mum wasn't well my stomach literally did flips and I felt sick. As soon as we got home I went straight up to Mum's room and asked her what was wrong. She had the flu. I asked her if I could do anything for her. She said no, that Nanny was seeing to dinner and making her a hot drink. I was so scared to go near her but so upset that she was ill. I didn't go downstairs and do my homework or watch TV like I usually would have done after school, I just stayed in my room with my door open so I could hear if Mum was OK.

My favourite TV shows were Michaela Strachan's animal programmes and Children's Hospital. I didn't relate the irony, and didn't necessarily relate the hospitals in the programmes to my own life but I just wanted to see what happened to people outside of the happy, colourful perception of normality that we are shown on TV as kids.

As I grew older, the feelings I experienced because of other people's emotions, and the feelings of dread that congealed in my stomach every time something was remotely upsetting, only grew stronger and I worried more. I worried about my grandparents living in a fairly rough area and constantly spoke to them about being careful around those teenagers and not to open the door to anyone and not to go out at night. I worried about animals being hurt every time I saw the animal programmes on TV and wondered how much it happened. I worried about money and my parents' financial struggle through life – this all before the age of seven. My parents never made me feel worried, I just picked up on anything that wasn't right. The worst or most profound example of my overwrought emotions was during the Gulf War of 1990-1991. My parents would speak to our family in Israel about air raids and bombs and war and danger and I sat listening to every phone conversation, trying to decipher my dad's language jumps from Hebrew to French to Arabic. The Arabic was so that I wouldn't understand, but I usually got the gist as it wasn't so dissimilar to Hebrew. Once the Gulf War had involved Israel, it was a huge part of the daily conversations in our house and it was always on the news. I didn't really understand what had happened to start the war but I understood that Israel, the United Kingdom and the United States were against the Iraqis, particularly, Saddam Hussein and that Saddam Hussein had no morals and didn't keep to the rules. I'd learned and could have spoken about Saddam Hussein, Margaret Thatcher, John Major, George H. W. Bush and Colin Powell. I was worried about Israel and about my family and I was worried about what would happen to the whole world if the war carried on. At the end of the war we got a call from my uncle to tell us they were all dancing in the street in Israel and had come out of their bomb shelters. I cried – actually cried – with happiness. Just to be clear, when the Gulf War broke out I was six years old.

I can't say that all this comes down to intelligence for we have established that although I wasn't as 'average' as people made out, I also wasn't the most intelligent. I think you can only put this frenetic intensity down to sensitivity. I was – and still am – way too sensitive and that makes life difficult. I see people who just aren't bothered by anything and they seem blissfully happy (unaware maybe?) in their lives of no feeling. Sometimes I wish I could be like them, other times I know that my awareness of other people's feelings makes me a better person because I can sympathise and empathise. It's the same way that now I talk and teach about a holistic approach to healthcare, some people think I'm mad because I'm not doing what the rest of society does, they're happy carrying on without knowing the truth. Sometimes I wish I was as blissfully unaware of truths that make life much harder. Mum bought me a book a few years ago called 'The Highly Sensitive Person'. After reading this book, all of a sudden my whole life made sense, not just to me but to everyone around me. I made Mum read the book herself so she could see and it has helped her understand me more. It explains that HSPs (highly sensitive person) make up about 15% of the population and although HSPs are affected by everything, without them the world would be a much worse place. Apart from HSPs being the ones who end up as carers, nurses etc and are just generally able to empathise and help out more (elderly people, animals, people with disabilities), apparently the best art comes from HSP's. The only people who can produce art to a level of believability – whether it be music, film, literature, artwork – are people who feel enough to translate it into their work. When you hear of musicians dying of overdoses and being drug addicts, they are usually the most talented ones (Amy Winehouse, Jimi Hendrix, Kurt Cobain, Billie Holiday, Jim Morrison – all the greats). They have too many emotions and feelings racing through their minds and it is impossible to deal with them all which is why many HSPs turn to drugs, to numb it down. I remember reading in Russell Brand's autobiography that even in his worst drug-addicted times when he lied and cheated and broke the law and got arrested, he never stopped being a vegetarian and always tried to help homeless people. I reckon he's an HSP, too. The Highly Sensitive Person is a great book. If you are relating to anything I just said, I highly recommend you read it.

Along with my over-wrought emotions, another characteristic was my sense of make-believe. I would concoct entire stories (some might call them lies) to make things more interesting. I once took an egg from the fridge, left it out in the garden covered by mud for a week so that it would look like a real bird's egg ready to hatch, then after that week I took it inside to Mum and told her that I found it in a bird's nest in the garden that must've fallen from a tree and the chick inside would now be unlikely to be reunited with its mother so we should look after it. She took one look at me, rolled her eyes and just said OK. I didn't know it then, but she knew when I was lying every single time.

I think a lot of the make-believe must have come from the books I read. I would get lost in Enid Blyton's whimsical world of wishing chairs and tree-houses and Roald Dahl's hilarious exaggeration on life. I grew into the Babysitter's Club and Sweet Valley High books (the original 'boxsets') – not the world's greatest literature but still enough to get my imaginative mind reeling with ideas. The Babysitter's Club made me decide that I didn't want to babysit but I could do the same as their club but with dog walking, which I did for about a week.

Despite my neurotic and intense approach to life, life did of course proceed, and it proceeded, arthritis first. Although I didn't mind leaving school for hospital appointments, I wasn't really sold on the podiatry clinic. The insoles were hideous – I hated them. I felt that they should have tried to make them more appealing to children. They were made of a deep mahogany brown leather-like material and smelt very odd. I didn't understand the need for them and would take them out of my shoes at any given opportunity but of course, my mum would always make me put them back in. Eventually, they did help, as my feet now have the arches they were missing for a few years.

There seemed to be a pattern with the illness. The Uveitis mainly flared up in June when the tree pollen count was high, but the joints would play up in the winter, when it was cold. On one occasion, when I was eight, I had a dreadful time with the ring finger on my left hand. I couldn't bend it properly and it just felt stuck. We saw Dr. Smith about it several times and, although I cannot remember what was said, I later asked Mum if I had arthritis in that hand. She became very upset, I remember – she hadn't realised that I didn't understand what was going on, after all doctors spoke to adults and not to children so I shouldn't have been expected to understand – and told me that if there was ever anything that I didn't understand about my arthritis, I should ask her. It turns out that I did have arthritis and it was in the tendon, which is what helps the finger to flex. I have never been able to bend that finger fully, although it helped me to learn my left from right. I knew the left hand was the affected one so whenever I had to figure out if something was left or right I'd clench my fists quickly to see which was the stiff one and know from that which way was left. So, I started to understand more, but the flare got worse. My knees and ankles were so swollen that I could barely move and I was given crutches by the physiotherapy team.

The only time that the crutches didn't worry me was one particular year during the Jewish festival of Shavuot. We all had to go to school dressed in white clothes with bright colours and the girls wore floral garlands in their hair. We put on shows for the parents in the assembly hall and, as Simi had sprained her ankle, she too had to sit on a chair, not on the floor with all the other children. It pleased me to be able to sit with a friend of mine for once, instead of next to a teacher. Simi was using her grandfather's very old-fashioned wooden walking stick, which I found funny. I told her that she looked like her Grandma.

We laughed at the fact that we were both invalids at the same time and for those few days I didn't mind having my crutches with me – I didn't feel so abnormal. Selfishly, I was disappointed when Simi's ankle improved and she didn't need the stick any more. I wondered if I would ever be better, or what it would be like to have a condition that just healed and got better.

After a month or so, my condition was not improving; in fact, it was getting worse. I was transferred to Great Ormond Street Children's Hospital in which Dr. Smith now held her clinic. The hospital was amazing – like a hotel for children. Every clinic was bursting with colour but in a different way from ordinary children's wards. It was clean, bright and modern and it didn't smell funny – this was the highlight for me. I was unable to eat in other hospitals because the smell of hospital food made me feel sick. Even if Mum brought in our own food, I still couldn't eat it while being around that hospital smell. Great Ormond Street didn't have that smell and I loved it.

Most clinics and all the wards had Nintendo computer games for children to play Super Mario Brothers on. There was just so much to do and that is why the hospital is such a success. Children feel happier there than in a normal hospital, as they are kept occupied by things that they want to do and not things they need to do and I'm sure this plays a vital part in getting better.

One day whilst visiting the hospital for a check-up, we had the most wonderful surprise. Princess Diana was due to visit and the hospital staff asked if I would like to meet her. Of course I wanted to meet her! Mum and I waited with all the other children and parents who were waiting to see her in the lobby. When she walked in, I was in awe. She was the most beautiful person I'd ever seen. She was wearing a mint green skirt suit and she was perfect. She walked past and shook each of our hands before making her way up to the wards. After she passed away – which was about four years after that – I was so happy that I had had the privilege of meeting her.

I was now seeing both Dr. Smith and Dr. Graham at Great Ormond Street so my joints and eyes could be treated in the same place. This suited me down to the ground as it removed the need for me to spend time in smelly hospital waiting rooms. During this particular flare-up, I received some steroid injections. I went into a rather inviting room on the lower ground floor of the Hospital with Mum and Nanny and was greeted by a very friendly South African doctor. He would be draining the fluid out of the five inflamed joints and then injecting steroid to control the inflammation. They did not usually treat so many joints at one time, but in my case there was so much fluid that they must have thought it best to remove it all at once.

I was given a sedative, which was injected through my hand. It made me very woozy, which was kind of nice, but I remember Mum sitting next to me on the bed holding my right hand – the one that wouldn't be injected - with her other arm under my head. Nanny sat in a chair in the opposite corner of the room. The doctor took over a pint of fluid from one knee and I remember that it was brown. Mum and I joked that it looked like Coca Cola. The doctor teased me by saying, "Be careful what you say, Lauren, because this medicine makes you tell the truth!" And so Mum asked me who I loved expecting I'd say her. Instead, I professed my love for a boy in year six (way too old for my current standing of year three) called Jonny.

Everyone started laughing. They finished draining that knee, as well as the other one, the two ankles and the left hand. I was well and truly exhausted.

Poppa did not come with us as he had become quite ill at this stage. Although I didn't know it at that time, he had prostate cancer and emphysema. He was a tall, broadly built man, with two fingers missing from an accident he'd had with a machine at the tobacco factory in which he used to work. My grandparents formed a huge part of my life and I couldn't imagine anything worse than losing them but, four months after my steroid injection nightmare, Poppa died in Edgware General Hospital. I had been to see him earlier that day and he told me that the people on the wall were moving and telling him to come towards them. The doctors said that he was hallucinating, but Mum and Nanny said they were the angels coming to take him to heaven.

My grandparents had belonged to a spiritual circle years before, and had instilled in us a strong belief in angels and life after death. I didn't know that he would die that day, but I think Mum did, because she took us home from the hospital and then went back there with her brother, Uncle Harry. Ilana and I were at home with Aba when Aunty Ruth (Uncle Harry's wife) called us. I remember bursting into tears and running upstairs when the phone rang and Aba picked up, and then I heard the words 'bad news'.

My Poppa would always sit and do my exercises with me, making them fun. He used to put me on his shoulders and bounce up and down. He bought me a rocking horse for my third birthday and carried it on his back, on buses, all the way from the East End to the suburbs. I still have Humphrey, that rocking horse, as it reminds me of Poppa. Mum said that he was never as good a father as he was a grandfather, and he was closer to us than he was to the other cousins but, to me, he was the world's best grandpa.

I wasn't allowed to go to the funeral, as I was too young, but I remember the people coming back to our house in the evening for prayers. Some of them were laughing and giggling and I didn't understand this. Even my cousin, Stacey, was laughing as if nothing had happened and this upset me, but she was older and I imagine that she was dealing with the loss in her own way.

I spent that day wondering who would now sit on the floor next to me and make me do the 'bicycle' exercise, saying 'hop, two, three, four... hop, two, three, four' and who would teach me inappropriate songs like 'Knees Up Mother Brown'. I also worried for Nanny because now she would be on her own. She stayed with us for a while but, after a month, she said that she should go home now or else she never would. She was a small, petite lady, always beautifully turned out, even when she was ill, and wore dangly earrings and beaded necklaces. She was fiercely independent and liked it that way. Her flat was only a five-minute drive from us, so it would be easy to see her.

A year before Poppa died, Nanny's best friend, Lily, also died and when this happened Nanny became really ill. To this day, we don't know what happened but, as soon as Aunty Lily died, Nanny developed some form of dysentery. She could not eat anything and had constant diarrhoea. She rapidly lost weight and, after Poppa died, it got worse. People in the street would stop and stare at her because she was so thin - it was scary. The next few months were bizarre, as the stress of everything had also made Mum quite ill. She became unable to move her neck and was in so much pain that she had to go to A&E, where they prescribed her some very strong painkillers. A few months later, Mum celebrated her 40th birthday and eventually started feeling a bit better, but ever since then, whenever she is stressed, she gets the same pain in her neck.

Safta - my grandmother in Israel – also died that year, so it was a very hard year for the whole family. We have never been a particularly religious family but, after Safta died, Aba went to Synagogue every Monday night for a year, to mourn. I don't know the significance of Monday nights, but he went every week without fail. We were not allowed to go with Aba to Israel for the funeral, but we visited the grounds a year later when Aba's brother got married.

Over the next few years, my health was extremely unstable. I was receiving weekly physio and hydro sessions, and steroid injections became a more regular occurrence which kind of countered the fact that Mum didn't want me to have oral steroids but she didn't have enough information and felt there was no other choice. The doctors told her there was no other choice. I think had I have been born in the internet age, Mum could have researched more, been part of online forums where other mums spoke to each other about treatment options but it was the early '90s and she did the best she could by taking me to the homeopath and controlling my diet in the only way she was taught but that was all the information she had so at times when I was at my worst, she had no option but to agree with the doctors. It took many years for us to get all the answers.

A few months before my tenth birthday, we received some good news. One of Mum's oldest friends, Lorraine, was now living in Florida and was working as a travel agent. She got us free flights and an amazing deal on the best hotel and we were going to Disney World!

We were so excited. Aba arranged for us to have new summer clothes to take with us, as we were dressed up for winter in London. We began to get ready for our big trip. But, as always, not everything went smoothly.

A few days before we were due to leave, my knees swelled so much that my legs looked like sticks with melons stuck through the middle. I could barely walk because they were so stiff and when I did, it felt as if there was jelly between my kneecaps and walking felt 'slushy'. As Dr. Smith did not have a clinic at Great Ormond Street on this particular day, we went to Northwick Park to see her, and she offered us two options; either I could have the fluid drained and steroid injected there and then, or I could wait until the following week and be booked in for sedation. But it was Friday and we were due to fly on the Monday. It was such a cruel choice for a nine year old to have to make but I knew what I had to do. When Mum asked me what I wanted to do, I decided to be brave and have the fluid drained while I was awake, as there was no way I was going to miss Disney World.

It is very hard to explain the feeling of having fluid drained from your body. I would have to say that at the age of nine, it was the most painful thing I had experienced up to that point and, even now, it is amongst the worst. Later on in my story, you will hear about the others.

I was put on a bed and numbing cream was applied over my knees, stuck on with a transparent sticky plaster that actually looked like my own skin wrinkling up. We had to wait about twenty minutes for the cream to work, but it seemed like a lifetime. Dr. Smith, albeit well regarded in her field, never really made me feel comfortable or calm – I think they call this a 'bedside manner'. Thankfully I had Mum there. She called Aba and told him to be ready to carry me up the stairs when we got home.

Just writing about draining the fluid makes my skin crawl. It is one thing having it done when you can't feel anything, but when you are nine years old and a huge needle is inserted into your knee and moved around inside, it is literally unbearable. If you can imagine having a large needle worming around inside you, sucking up fluid until there is no more left, that is what it's like. I didn't know how long it would take for all the fluid to be drained and, meanwhile, I could do nothing but squirm and cry while having to sit still and wait for it to be over. Aside from that, the worst thing about the whole process was that once one knee had been done, I knew what was coming with the other one, which made it harder to cope with and I was crying like a baby. I had always been told that I was quite brave but on this particular day I felt anything but brave.

Both knees were drained and injected with steroid and somehow I got through it. Mum made me a promise that she would never let me go through that again. We would later find out that this promise was unfortunately one that was impossible to keep.

We did however board the plane on Monday and enjoyed the best holiday a child could wish for. The plane journey was a struggle in itself, before we'd even arrived. The limited space was a problem for me, as I needed to stretch my legs out to avoid them getting stiff. I tried to stretch them across my parents' laps but, after about five hours of trying to keep quiet, it was too much. I was crying because of the pain. Aside from the throbbing pain of the actual arthritis, the tenderness from the injections was still very evident and difficult to ignore on an eight-hour flight. Eventually we arrived and were met at the airport by a very friendly American with a wheelchair, who would be helping my parents to push me to the Arrivals area.

Because of the amount of walking round the theme parks, we hired a pushchair, which was supposed to be for Ilana. Mum and Aba contemplated hiring a wheelchair for me, but I refused. Instead, poor Ilana ended up walking everywhere, because I took her place in the pushchair. I just couldn't walk around for that amount of time after the ordeal my knees had just been through.

In Disney World, there were all sorts of people. Older children in pushchairs, children in wheelchairs and older people in what looked like prams, so I didn't feel that different and wasn't too bothered about sitting in a pushchair. Had it have been in London, I would have worried about people staring but, here, I was having such a nice time that I didn't want to ruin the memories by walking too much and suffering later – so the pushchair it was. The great thing is that, in spite of what I had been through a few days before we arrived, none of my memories from that holiday are of being in pain. I remember sitting in the pushchair to prevent the pain, but I don't recall actually being in pain as such.

Chapter 4

The Transition

Less than two years after visiting Disney World, I turned eleven and started secondary school. I chose JFS in Camden Town.

Children from Rosh Pinah who were exceptionally clever went on to private schools, one of which being the City Of London School for Girls, which is where Simi went, firstly because she was clever and secondly because it was a girls' school and her mum didn't want her to be distracted by boys. Rachel went to Emmanuel College, a private Jewish school and generally for those whose parents had money. The rest of us, in fact, most of my class from Rosh Pinah, went to JFS so I wasn't alone.

The journey to school in itself was a challenge. Before starting secondary school, I had never been allowed to get on a bus or train on my own and now I would be catching two buses and a train every morning, just to get there.

The first bus was from near my house to Edgware Station and this part of the journey I would have to make on my own but once I arrived at Edgware, I would greet the pool of Smurfs (our uniforms were royal blue) that congregated there, all waiting for each other to catch the train together.

Luckily, in spite of there being eight classes in the one year group, my friend Miranda and I were put into the same class which was a bonus. JFS seemed a huge place to us, as we had come from such a small school where we knew everyone's names. All of a sudden, we were faced with two thousand pupils, a huge bunch of teachers whose names we thought we'd never remember and a gigantic building. Like a troop of chameleons, we soon adapted.

On my first day of school, I stood outside my house with my long wavy hair just perfect, not one hair out of place, wearing my royal blue sweatshirt with a baby blue shirt underneath and a grey pleated skirt. Mum took a picture of me holding my school bag. It appears that I started out as a real geek at school. Mum had bought Miranda and me Carlton rucksacks to use as school bags as they were 'sturdy and safe for our backs'. After a few years we would never have chosen something because of how 'sturdy' it was. It was all about Kookai record bags decorated with markers and Tipex. My skirt was also much longer than I like to remember. We were told that girls had to wear their skirts at a 'modest' length. I didn't want to get told off on my first day so my pleated skirt was just below my knees and my brand new black leather school shoes from Clarks were still quite childlike. It took all of about a month to realise that I had to pull it together and ditch the lumpy navy jacket, the Carlton school bag and the long skirt.

I met Loredana, or Lolly, in Year 7, soon after I started at JFS. She wasn't in any of my classes but we met on the train and just clicked.

Lolly and I actually looked quite similar. We both had long dark hair and olive skin and were about the same shape and height. She was less of a girly girl than I was and laughed at how I constantly arranged my fringe to look perfect and how I carried around a tiny eyebrow brush to perfect my eyebrows brushed my eyebrows so that they would be straight. She suggested that I grow my fringe out like she did and then I wouldn't have to keep playing with it. The quest for perfection continued.

At twelve years old and living in the suburbs of London, you rely on your parents to take you everywhere. When this was not possible and there was nowhere to go, Lolly and I found ways to keep ourselves occupied. When we were at her house, we were outdoors all the time and played with her neighbours.

There was a field next to Lolly's house and we often donned wellington boots and high socks – to avoid being stung by the nettles – and searched for weird and wonderful creatures. For some reason, we genuinely believed that we would find snakes and scorpions in the middle of a farm field in Harrow. Lolly was usually happy to just sit and watch TV, but I was somewhat adventurous and would drag her along to participate in my adventurous games, which, after much persuasion, she enjoyed in the end.

Mum had taught me a game called 'Have A Cigarette, Sir', - appropriate, I know. We cut a pair of tights in half to make two 'legs', put a tennis ball in one of them and tied this leg up. I then stood with my back against the outside wall of my house, holding the leg of the tights that had the ball in it in my right hand and knocking it from my right side to my left, while singing the song 'Have A Cigarette, Sir'. At the word 'Sir', I lifted a leg and knocked the ball under my leg onto the wall. Eventually, Lolly caught on and we would then compete to see who could finish quicker without forgetting to lift a leg. This game kept us occupied for hours on end and I wonder if we'd had iPads and video games and computers in those days if I would have come away with as many funny memories.

One day when we were twelve years old, sitting on the bus on the last leg of our long journey to school, a man of around fifty years old, dirty and unkempt, stood in front of us while we sat on the seats at the front of the bus. He was holding on to a railing to keep himself up and we thought nothing of it, surely he was just trying to keep from falling over and that is why he was so close. But with no warning, the man put his hand on my knee. I froze. I remember simply freezing and not knowing what to do as he edged his hand further and further up my skirt. I couldn't even move my eyes or take a breath, I didn't know what to do and my mind wasn't even thinking quickly enough to be able to gauge whether or not this was wrong. We never had the talks and lectures from our parents in those days about sexual activity and what to look out for, I suppose our parents didn't even consider it. As his hand reached right up to the top of my thigh, Lolly shouted, "Take your hand off my friend's leg!" He did, and we arrived at the bus stop outside school around twenty seconds later where Lolly had to grab me and drag me out of the bus. She took me straight to the security office where she explained exactly what had happened, like a protective mother, bless her. I was still silent, in shock I suppose. The security team called the police and my parents, and Aba came to the school straight away as did Lolly's parents. Aba tried to act normal and not too angry or worried. The police asked me to describe the man which I did once I'd regained composure and once they left I simply said to Aba, "Well, if I'm getting the day off school, can I go to Lolly's??" I didn't get the significance of what happened at twelve years old and maybe that was a good thing.

Between the ages of twelve and sixteen, the arthritis stayed reasonably stable. The doctors had said that it was probably 'burning out', which they said commonly happens when children reach their teenage years. I didn't have more than one flare-up a year and it was rare that my knees and ankles were swollen or uncomfortable. I still had to be monitored at hospital fairly regularly and would occasionally turn up at school bearing a crutch, but I don't remember it happening too much. I really don't remember the arthritis affecting my teenage years very much at all.

My adolescence, as with everyone, was a funny old time. The summer of 1997, when I was thirteen and a half, my periods started. Normally this would have been fine, it was expected. What I didn't expect was for my dad to come in from work and into my room and exclaim, "Lauren! Mazal tov!" I was mortified and couldn't understand what possessed my mum to tell him. Could nothing be a secret? That's when you know when you're a teenager; not when your periods start but when you want to start being secretive about anything and everything, when you start locking your door and are constantly moody and want no one to talk to you or ask you questions. That attitude pretty much began that very same day.

That same summer I went to Israel on my own for the first time. I stayed with Uncle Asher and Aunty Zahava in their mad house, which was still buzzing with as many people as it had when we were kids. Anyone who was visiting from abroad stayed with them.

I was picked up from the airport by my cousin Oren, who was eighteen at the time and, as I landed at 5:30 in the morning, he was on his way back from clubbing. We arrived at the house when everyone was still sleeping – and there were people everywhere. I wasn't too impressed with the mess, but I unpacked my case and went to sleep.

It was the first time that I had been away from my parents and I think it did me good. I was still a child but something changed in me once I returned from that holiday – I had made the transition from child to teenager.

When I went back to school in the September, I felt completely different and started doing older things. I became much more interested in boys, and one in particular. His name was Ben and he was two years older than me. At the time, it seemed to be much more than a crush; I genuinely believed that I was in love with him. I would sit in the playground at lunchtime, staring at him and doodling his name over my books. I even took photographs of him that I kept in my diary so that I could stare at his face during lessons.

During this year, Miranda and I started to drift apart and I found new friends, often from outside the Rosh Pinah group. Lolly and I were still very close, but she had also started to make new friends and, although we were still friendly with each other, we acquired our own separate friendship groups.

I had met Charlotte (Charlie) a few months before. She was from Southgate and I had never really spoken to her before, as the Southgate kids kept to themselves, much as the Edgware group did. Charlie was, and still is, one of the funniest people I have ever met.

She was completely different from Lolly. Most of the Southgate kids were quite naughty, or at the very least, cheeky, and Charlie was no exception – she was cheeky in a way that was endearing, as was her best friend, Oniel – whom every girl in the year fancied, me included. Lolly was always scared to get into trouble or do anything slightly adventurous, whereas Charlie was up for anything and adventures appealed to me.

Charlie and I adopted this stupid accent which we used whenever we had something funny to say and it made the story we were telling sound even funnier. When I was with Charlie, all we did was laugh. Everything was funny and if it wasn't, we'd make it funny.

Charlie and I did everything together. I liked the way that she would sit in the playground with me at lunchtimes, watching the older boys playing football while we listened to Backstreet Boys, A1 and Mariah Carey on my Walkman. I hoped that Ben would pay attention to me sitting there – of course he never did. In fact, he was so aware of my obsession that he would try to get away from me whenever he could – poor sod.

I had decided to take my Hebrew GCSE two years early in a private establishment outside school. For GCSE, we were only allowed to choose one language and I was getting on so well with French that I wanted to continue but it seemed silly to miss the opportunity to get a high grade in Hebrew so I did Hebrew outside of school in Year 9. The lessons were quite expensive, so I had to give up my guitar lessons. Once I took my last lesson, I didn't pick up a guitar again. Other distractions were taking up all my time. Mum was really upset and tried to convince me to practice again, but I never did. What a waste of seven years of hard work, dedication and very expensive weekly lessons. Why do teenagers have to be such hard work??

Something clicked in me during this school year and I realised how much of my childhood had revolved around my illness. As a child, you accept the hand you are dealt because you know no different; you learn to live with it and adapt, but now, after meeting so many new people at school, I could see for the first time how different I was and how unusual my childhood had been, and I resented it.

Now that the arthritis was finally stable, it was the first time in my life that I had distractions other than hospitals, homeopaths, injections and hydro pools, and I savoured every moment. This realisation led me to want to take control of my life which, in turn, made me become completely obsessive and controlling.

I obsessed over Ben to the point of insanity and I stopped eating. I saw food as something I had complete control over and no one could stop that. Whether or not the arthritis flared again, food was the one thing I could control. I also wanted to look perfect. I started blow-drying my hair every day to make it dead straight (all the rage in the '90s) and spent all my pocket money on finding a concealer that would cover up the damn dark circles that had resided under my eyes since I was two. Every break time, I would take out my concealer and mirror and re-apply some more, so that there was no evidence of those ugly, dark bags that were constant reminders of the pain.

I spent the majority of that year drinking a Mars milkshake in the morning on the way to school, as I thought it would give me enough energy to last the day and then I'd eat an apple for lunch, and take it straight to the playground so I could see Ben, instead of wasting time in the lunch hall. Charlie and I would sit there listening to our music, gossiping, sketching pictures on our school books and, of course, staring not so discreetly at our crushes.

By May, I had lost so much weight that my head looked too big for my body and my bones, especially the collar and hip bones, were protruding and skeleton-like. I had gone from being a chubby eleven year-old with Miranda, to an average twelve year-old with Lolly, to a ridiculously skinny thirteen year-old, all because of a boy and a resentment towards my illness. I didn't notice the weight loss myself, which was bizarre bearing in mind that it had dropped so quickly.

One day, my parents had some friends over for a barbeque and when one of Mum's friends, Rosi, looked at me in shock and blurted out, "Lauren, why are you so thin? What happened?" I was delighted and examined myself in the mirror, but couldn't see anything different to how I had always been. I grabbed my belly and convinced myself that it was too wobbly and there was too much of it. I wondered what on earth Rosi was talking about, but I was still happy that someone thought I looked thin. I have two pictures from that time and both show me to look severely underweight, it's actually scary.

For some reason, starving myself came quite naturally to me. I didn't seem to need too much food to exist and I surprised myself at how long I could go without feeling hungry. This made it a lot easier, as it didn't hurt and it was fun to see how long I could control my hunger.

I had spent the past nine months arguing with my parents because they didn't understand what was going through my head. They would force me to eat dinner every night, but some nights I got away with it, or at least I got away with eating as little as possible.

One day, without warning, one of my friends stepped in and told Mum that I was starving myself. Nicola was a friend of mine from school but our mothers were friendly too and so she thought that it was right to say something. Ironically enough, Nicola ended up suffering with bulimia as she got older. Mum had tried to reason with me many times before this, but that particular night she angrily confronted me, when it was just the two of us alone in the lounge. She was crying, telling me how she'd always done so much to keep me healthy and now I was ruining it all by making myself ill. When she said that, something in me clicked. I felt guilty and sad for her. This woman sitting in front of me, crying, had literally spent the last fourteen years doing everything in her power to keep me well and here I was, throwing it all back in her face with my treacherous, unjustified behaviour. I just couldn't do that. I cried with her, gave her a hug, apologised for being so selfish and made myself a hot chocolate before going to bed.

I don't know why it was so easy for me to snap out of it. Perhaps my mum meant more to me than gaining back the control I felt I'd lacked and although it was labelled as an eating disorder, it wasn't really that, because eating disorders are things that people battle with their whole lives. I have always been body conscious, but have never lapsed back into that way of life since that day. I just craved the control and once I realised that I had that control in my life, I was able to let it go.

After that, I had to eat my lunches in the medical room for a few months to be monitored, but that too, soon passed. I also ate breakfast and dinner and didn't complain.

Ben soon took his GCSEs and left school, but I had lost interest by this point. I had moved on from whatever it was that I was looking for through being obsessed with someone. Once I got some perspective, I was embarrassed by just how obsessed I had been. My friends all had crushes on boys, but none of them were ever as obsessed as I had been with Ben. If you're reading this, sorry Ben! You know who you are. I'm not crazy I promise! (Well, maybe a little.)

Perhaps I had needed a distraction that took up all of my time, so that I could think about nothing else. I had certainly achieved that, but messed up so many other things in the process. My friendships revolved around my eating – or lack thereof – and my parents didn't trust me, so I had to fix this.

I made a decision there and then to never become obsessed with a man again and I am glad that I learned this lesson at the age of fourteen. It would not, however, be the last time a man would have that kind of hold over me.

The school year came to an end and the looming summer was once again upon us but mine wasn't to be a summer of fun as I had to have my tonsils removed, so we didn't have a holiday abroad.

I always remembered the more affluent kids talking about their summers in Marbella, and I wondered what this mystical land of Marbella might look like. At the time, these kids seemed so rich compared to me that I imaged Marbella as you might imagine the Maldives; white sandy beaches, turquoise water, hoola girls and flower necklaces (yes, I know that is more Hawaii, but Hawaii and the Maldives could have been two cities in Japan for all I knew.)

After recovering from my tonsillectomy, Mum took us for a week's break to the Isle of Wight. Nanny came with us and we stayed in a huge caravan on a campsite. Everyone was watching everything I ate which got a bit tedious at times, but we had a good time and I managed to leave Year 9 behind me.

When we arrived back home, I had a letter waiting for me with my Hebrew GCSE result. I had managed to pass with A*. I was relieved that my rebellion hadn't gone so far as to affect my grades and once the feeling of relief passed, I was very happy with myself.

The following school year I was a lot happier, but I got up to quite a bit of mischief. For some reason, no matter what I did at school, I was never caught and very rarely got into trouble. Yes, I know what you're thinking; one of those annoying ones. I don't know why, but most of the teachers seemed to like me, with the exception of my science teacher, Mr. Brigham, who sent me out of the class on numerous occasions for disrupting the lesson by throwing Jelly Tots and trying to get them to land in his bum-bag.

By now, because we were in GCSE mode, the classes were more mixed and we didn't have classes purely with people from our own house. This suited me, as it meant I had some classes with Lolly. She sat next to me in science and found my Jelly Tot throwing very amusing, although she was far too scared of getting into trouble herself to ever consider throwing sweets at a teacher.

Mr. Brigham was a prime target for children intent on terrorising a teacher. He bore an uncanny resemblance to Harold Bishop from Neighbours, and was known as 'Jelly Belly', with his low drooping, chubby cheeks and balding head. His daily choice of outfit consisted of a claret red velvet blazer and a bum-bag, and his first name was Crispin. I mean, come on! He really couldn't really have made it any easier for us. I would greet him at the start of every lesson with the song

'Smelly Cat' – as sung by Phoebe in Friends – with the words 'smelly cat' changed to 'Brigi-bums'. Highly immature, I know but, at fifteen years old, the rest of the class were amused by it and I enjoyed being thought of as funny. Mr Brigham would threaten to write our names on the board if we were naughty, but this name-writing never amounted to anything so we were pretty much able to be as badly behaved as we liked. On rare occasions, we would be sent to sit outside the office of one of the three Deputy Head Teachers. I was always sent to Ms. Hamnett and the routine was the same every time. She would look at me in disgust, tell me to stop disrupting Mr. Brigham's class, write a bad note in my diary, and then hand over a bottle of acetone and some cotton wool and I would remove my nail varnish. This happened about once every two months.

Lolly sat to my right in science lessons, on the second bench from the front, with Sophie (yup, same one from nursery) and Judy to the right of Lolly and two boys called Duncan and David who sat to my left. David entertained us during the humdrum of Photosynthesis by showing us his 'party-trick'. This consisted of him resting a ruler on his penis – over the top of his trousers, in case you were worried that it was tasteless and bordering on underage something-or-other – and demonstrating how he could move the ruler up and down using only that part of his body. Most of the boys seemed to love this trick and a few of them did have the gumption to actually perform it with the trouser zip open, unlike David who was kind enough not to reveal his genitals. None of us girls were that impressed, but we went along with it anyway, I'm not sure why.

Fifteen year-old boys must have a great deal of pent-up sexual frustration, as I cannot explain the amount of penis-touching we witnessed during classes. Only the ones we referred to as sluts – and there were many of them – would engage in these activities with the boys, but the rest of us just watched on in awe.

Although David spent much time perfecting his penis/ruler demonstration, he had other talents too. He spent the majority of the lesson humming songs to himself, but not as quietly as he thought. His favourite was a rendition of Wonderful Tonight and when he hummed this one, we all sang along. At the same time, Duncan would sit bopping his head to the music coming out of his Discman earphones, shouting at Mr. Brigham whenever he was asked to turn off the music. Our science class was more of a circus show. Lolly, Sophie and Judy used to observe all this, laughing hysterically as I threw Jelly Tots into Mr. Brigham's bum-bag, but were all far too scared of getting into trouble to ever be less than subtle about it. They would spend most of the lesson discussing Lolly's three-year-long crush on a boy called Joe. So, quite worryingly, not much studying was actually done.

I don't know why I was less scared than they were at getting in trouble, but we were very different characters. I didn't ever want to get into serious trouble, so I never did anything awful, (well, apart from blocking the sinks in every toilet and flooding the school so we got sent home, but that's another story altogether) but I liked to have fun and didn't want to take things too seriously. I was just enjoying myself, acting my age and not having a care in the world.

Lolly has since said that some of her funniest memories are from those days in science class. Apart from anything, it gave us something to talk about after class other than Bunsen burners and the Periodic Table.

I bunked off lessons too. Probably more than I should have done. (Well, how much should one really bunk off lessons?) A few of us had discovered a disused toilet, which hadn't been used since the 1970s and no one, not even the teachers, knew about it. We named it 'the black room', as it was unlit and pitch black.

We got up to all sorts of mischief in the black room. The girls would flirt with the boys by sitting on their laps (there were not enough chairs and it was difficult to smuggle more in without being seen) and, sometimes, couples would go into the cubicles and indulge in some snogging action, perhaps some indulged in some more action.

One day, when we were supposed to be in our post-lunch lesson, Danielle, Oniel, Oniel's friend Jonny and I all stayed in the black room to bunk the lesson and after about ten minutes of talking and flirting, the boys suggested that we go into the cubicles – Jonny with me and Danielle with Oniel. I was really nervous. I'd kissed some boys at parties, but this was less public and I didn't know what Jonny expected of me. He was very popular and had been with a lot of girls and I was worried that I wouldn't be experienced enough for his liking. As I started kissing Jonny, I found it very enjoyable. I had butterflies in my stomach and enjoyed the feeling of being wanted, but it didn't take too long for Jonny to insinuate that he wanted more by trying to push my head down towards his lap. I was hugely offended and way more naïve than I gave myself credit for, and after grabbing Danielle from the neighbouring cubicle, I ran out of the black room – not able to go anywhere as it was still lesson time. We hid in the ground floor toilets until we heard the bell for the next lesson. Danielle and I laughed about it, but I couldn't face Jonny for months after that.

I had had my first kiss the year before, when I was thirteen, at a party for under-16s. The boy was called Josh and we shared a few classes at school. At thirteen and about to have my first kiss, I was not only very nervous but also uncomfortably aware that everyone was watching. As I sat on a bench tilting my head in preparation for the biggest moment of my life thus far, and hoping that I wouldn't make a complete mess of it, we realised that we had an audience of about twenty friends who believed that it was normal to watch. Apparently, it was. I don't think I messed it up in the end, but it was a bizarre experience. All I could think about was whether or not I was doing it right – this is not something that your parents, or even your friends, can teach you. You just pray to God that you are breathing out of your nose, not your mouth, that your breath doesn't smell and that he won't go back and tell his friends that you don't know how to kiss.

This first kiss was monumentally significant for me at the time. Well, they usually are, aren't they, otherwise we wouldn't remember who it was with.

While bunking in the black room, we would also smoke cigarettes and some of the boys smoked weed in there. Most of the pupils got into trouble for not showing up to class, but I must have had some sort of good girl image that led the teachers to think that I would never get up to anything naughty and so they believed my stories of why I hadn't been present. Either that or they felt sorry for me. Only two teachers didn't like me – the Head of Year and my science teacher – the latter quite understandably.

The Head of Year called me into her office on a daily basis, to tell me that my skirt was too short and I was wearing too much jewellery. Of course, the minute I left her office, I would roll my skirt back up and put my jewellery back on.

Another place we would go when bunking off was the boiler room, where we would sit and speak to the maintenance men who didn't seem to mind us being there.

By Year 11, the security guards found out about the black room and boarded it up. As if that was going to stop us! The black room was situated by the entrance to the back playground and was separated from the school by a small stone staircase, under which was another 'room', painted orange. We made this room our little project and, between 10 of us, transformed it from the 'orange room' to the 'green room'. It became the green room for two reasons: firstly, because we didn't like the colour, so we painted it green (the very clever and overly observant security guards who took six months to discover the black room, had failed to notice a bunch of fifteen year olds bringing tins of paint into school) and, secondly, because of all the green that was smoked in there. I tried it a few times, but was always scared that I wouldn't make it home in one piece if I got really stoned, so I would casually turn down the spliff being passed around the room whilst aiming to maintain an utterly cool image.

One of my classic trouble-causing moments was after Jonny and I started talking again and we teamed up to stage the infamous JFS Lunch Strike. We wanted to draw attention to the fact that our lunches cost too much, but we also wanted to have a bit of fun. We managed to convince most of our year group – other than the obvious geeks who never wanted to get into trouble – to join in. We made banners and brought in whistles and musical instruments, and as lunchtime began on this particular day, Jonny and I spread the word.

Twenty teenagers stood in the lunch hall holding up banners, jumping on the tables and chanting, while the rest of us positioned ourselves in the middle playground – at exactly the point where everyone walked through to get to their classes after lunch – and also started chanting. We even managed to convince the younger pupils to get involved and chant with us. Ilana had just started at the school, so she persuaded her friends to join in and they all thought Ilana's older sister was, like the coolest.

After about forty-five minutes, in an unexpected turn of events, the police appeared and took some of the boys up to the Deputy Headmaster's office. For some reason, I was merely told to go to class, which I think annoyed a few of the boys and actually, it annoyed me too. It was my strike, my baby. The beginning of my anti-establishment days, the start of my as yet unknown road towards non-conformism and I should have got the credit for it. In the end I did. The story made it into the Jewish Chronicle, naming Jonny and me as the instigators and I was very proud of myself for causing a stir and making people aware of something that they clearly needed to be made aware of. Mostly, we were all very proud of ourselves for causing so much commotion that the whole Jewish community now knew about it.

The lunch prices were not reduced, however, so my efforts were futile but not utterly futile. It gave me a taste of things to come.

At some point during my penultimate school year, the school decided to implement a class council type thing, where one student from each class (eight classes per year, five main school years plus two sixth form years) would be elected as council leader and I thought I'd try my luck at it.

One day during chemistry – which I enjoyed way more than biology with Mr. Brigham because Mr. Dawes, our chemistry and physics teacher was great and I enjoyed blowing things up and watching things change composition – a tannoy went off right in the middle with the deputy head announcing each council leader for the whole school. "10AH, Lauren Vaknine," he said, I think somewhat shocked himself. I was very happy with myself, and during lunchtime registration that same day I took it upon myself to go around the class asking my fellow students what changes they would like to see implemented. I wrote everything down in my notebook like a 1920s New York reporter and set off to change the world with revolutionary ideas about how a school should be run. I liked the idea of leading a group, of speaking for the people and of organising change.

We met with our fellow council leaders once a month in the sixth form block (which I'd never previously been in before) and we were led by the sixth form leaders. We were split into our houses; Angel, Brodetsky, Weitzman and Zangwill. There were two classes per year in each house, so with all the years it worked out to four sets of fourteen people. My house was Angel, and on our first meeting the sixth form leaders went around the table asking us all about our ideas. "10AH?" Said the sixth form girl, who had massive boobs. She made me wonder if it was just a case of waiting three years until I was her age, and then I'd have boobs like that. No, it turns out that not everyone has boobs like that at eighteen years old, but I was fixated on how hers got so big. "Right," I said. "I think we should be able to have more choice in which subjects we pick for GCSE. What if I want to take History *and* Geography? And why should my parents have had to pay for me to take Hebrew privately outside of school? Why couldn't I have done Hebrew early *within* the school and still have taken French? There should be some sort of system for bilingual students to benefit from their abilities," I continued. "What about drama? We don't even offer drama and are completely uninspired in the arts. I've barely picked up a recorder let alone an actual instrument in the four years I've been here. Where's the music? What am I going to do with Pythagoras Theorem and Algebra when I leave school? I'm never going to be a scientist or a mathematician," I was getting angry now. "I mean, seriously, the pupils who are not good at academic subjects should be encouraged in things they can do. Teachers should be finding their strengths, not belittling them for their weaknesses because they can't remember every element on the periodic table. Things need to change!" "Lauren," said the power-hungry but somewhat perplexed sixth former. "We're not here to change the entire education system! You'll have to speak to the Government. Right, back to a proposed tuck shop..." And that is where it began; my need to be involved in change, in reforming systems that no longer worked and served only a few, in being a part of ideas that would change the world by speaking up for the masses, the ones who suffered but didn't know it, questioning the things that no one ever questioned because the masses are led by governments and large corporations to believe that things are the way they are meant to be. But they aren't the way they are meant to be, they are there to serve the 1% and as I got older I would become more involved in this idea, and more passionate in my quest for change in everything from the education system, to the food industry, to the dreaded pharmaceutical industry. Things that run the world but everyone trusts because they have no choice, but in the end, can they really be trusted? My fifteen year old self seemed to be the only one interested in the bigger picture and what also began in that sixth form block that day was my frustration at everyone else for not caring about change, about revolution. I was frustrated at them for not wanting to see beyond the tuck shop and the unimportant, trivial matters that would change absolutely nothing other than their waistlines. I would forever be frustrated with people for not understanding the importance of my missions, and for thinking me weird for wanting such colossal change, but in truth, I found out later on in life that despite the perpetual inadequacies of 'the system', all anyone ever really cared about was the proverbial tuck shop. It would be a hard lesson for me that anyone who ever really succeeded in changing things were the people who were dismissed as crazy for years first, people who were labelled as 'too extreme' or 'anti-convention' or 'anti-establishment' or, more commonly these days, 'hippie'. I'm not anti-establishment, I just think the establishment isn't run properly! So anyway, everyone around that table agreed that the tuck shop was the main priority, mostly because tuck shops are a privilege lost on Jewish schools because of the strict Kashrut laws. For them, this could be revolutionary in itself, but in truth, all it would do was create fatter kids. And trust me, Jewish kids never went hungry.

Lauren the Revolutionary to the side for a minute – or another few years – school continued and I worked hard in the subjects I actually liked, and worked less hard in the subjects I didn't, which is probably the reason I was always labelled as just 'average' in a scholastic sense of the word.

I especially loved English and adored my English teacher, Miss Ainley. Like I pointed out earlier, the state school system is not set up in a way to bring the best out of all children. They do not push us to find our vocation, our passion or what we are really good at. We are encouraged away from the arts and towards things that will have no relevance to us later on. I mean, what sort of school doesn't offer drama?? Had someone have taken the time to figure me out, they would have extracted a few hidden truths within me: I was interested in drama, English and history. But I was pushed so deeply into the wrong direction that when having to choose between history and geography for GCSE, the teacher told me to choose geography because she said I'd find the exam easier and I wasn't clever enough for the history exam. There was no one there saying, 'but hey, wait a minute, you're good at history and you enjoy it, let's explore this.' No one cared. Apart from two teachers.

There are some teachers who have a knack of making children like them – especially the naughty ones – and, if teachers can endear themselves to the naughtier elements, then the rest of the class will follow suit. This was the case both with Miss Ainley and also Miss Grodzinski, our Jewish Studies teacher.

Miss Grod, as we called her, got a grip on our very naughty, loud class and taught us in a way that got everyone interested. Every Wednesday, she would bring us bagels at lunchtime and instead of going to the lunch halls, we would join her in her classroom and eat lunch, while asking questions about Judaism. This is how we learnt, and this is how I achieved A grades in GCSE English and GCSE Jewish Studies. I got A* in both Hebrew and French, and everything else was a C and maths, of course, was a D. I got the A grades in the subjects that had good, inspiring teachers, and A* in languages that my parents had taught me. It gives some credit to home schooling, wouldn't you say?

Miss Ainley and Miss Grodzinski were the only teachers who managed to get me to enjoy learning again. One piece of English coursework that I had to do just before sitting my GCSEs was on racism and slavery in the Deep South. This was a subject that I had always been passionate about and so I wrote the piece effortlessly. Miss Ainley said that it was one of the best pieces of writing she had ever seen from a student of my age and I was extremely proud of myself. I managed to find a subject matter that I was passionate about and to this day I still read a lot about the history of slavery and the history of America and I believe that had there have been more teachers like Miss Ainley, I possibly would have achieved more earlier on.

My last two years of school were amongst the best years of my life. At lunchtimes, Charlie and I had moved ourselves to a different playground and found some other boys (still older than us) to watch. Much more docile and innocent than it had been with Ben, but it was still fun.

We spent our weekends going to Capital At Home, which was a live music show on a Saturday afternoon run by Capital Radio. All the top pop acts of the moment would perform every week and somehow we won tickets for months on end.

Saturday nights would be spent at friends' houses, the Finchley Lido Cinema complex, hanging around Golders Green and at parties. I stopped feeling like something was missing and just felt like a normal teenager who hung out with friends and had fun.

I met Gemma along the way, on one of our nights out at some under 16 disco. She went to Mill Hill County and I suppose it was nice to socialise with people other than the ones we saw every day. We became friends and remain friends to this day. Gemma was short and petite, with long blonde hair and blue eyes – she was every teenage boy's dream, they all loved her and made her a conquest. She was short, petite and blonde. I was tall, lanky and dark. I was beginning to learn an important lesson about what makes men's heads turn...

Hospital appointments were not as regular throughout high school – maybe once a month – and I was able to do most of the things that my friends could. I say most things, because there were a few that I could not do. I was completely useless at anything sports-related and I dreaded PE lessons. I had absolutely no co-ordination when it came to sports. Netball was the only game I half- enjoyed, but I was hopeless at it and so no one threw me the ball. If they did, I couldn't get it into the net without hitting myself in the face with it first. Mum said not to take it to heart, because I had an excuse, but it was still embarrassing and I sometimes wondered if there was anyone else as clumsy and uncoordinated as I was.

Luckily for me there was, and she came in the form of my best friend, Charlie. If anything, she was actually clumsier than me. Once, she fell into a rubbish bin while lining up outside our French class. I'm not quite sure how she even managed this but manage it she did. Charlotte's clumsiness gave me some confidence back. We laughed at all our stupid misfortunes and had fun with it. Before her, I just used to be embarrassed at myself for all my physical inadequacies and now my self-esteem was growing; only slightly but still growing.

The only sport that I ever enjoyed was trampolining. I had always been a bit of an adrenaline junkie – I liked heights, was the only person I knew who enjoyed turbulence on planes and I liked speed – so jumping as high as I could on a trampoline appealed to me. We learned how to manoeuvre ourselves into different positions, such as sitting, star jumps and somersaults. The PE teacher said that if enjoyed it that much, I should join the trampolining class on Tuesday lunchtimes. I tried to convince Charlie to join me, but she decided that it was not a good idea for her to be jumping anywhere where there was not a rail for her to hold on to.

I started going to the classes every Tuesday lunchtime and at my next appointment with Dr. Smith I told her all about my new found love of sport. To my disappointment, she told me that trampolining was too much for my knees to take and would damage my knees and I should stop immediately. That was the first and last sport that I enjoyed until my late twenties because I had been led to believe by a woman who should have been promoting exercise for health, that it was bad for me. Yet another example of authoritative figures conditioning our minds into believing something which is not only completely false but will also be more than detrimental to our well-being in the long-run. Her negative attitude and response to my enjoyment of this sport made me give up on anything physical at all. My doctor had told me that exercise was bad and I was fifteen, so I believed her and that was it for about ten years.

Once a year, in PE, we had to do the Beep Test, which was a test of physical ability and stamina - clearly something I was looking forward to (!) The PE teacher played a tape upon which a voice would say '1', '1.1', '1.2', '1.3' and it would increase in speed as the numbers went on. Between each number, we had to run the length of the playground. Charlie and I reached a maximum of 2, but would usually drop out before that, completely out of breath and unable to talk. The teacher shouted at us, telling us to stop being so lazy and carry on, but we just laughed and Charlie said, in a completely uninterested tone, "Sorry Miss, she's got arthritis and I'm on my period – we can't really be assed." With that, we would sit on the wall and chat and hope that it would be over soon, so that we could eat lunch.

Unfortunately, we had to wait for Abigail – a professional athlete in our year – to finish the whole Beep Test. She refused to quit until she got to the end. Her friends, who had finished a while before her and had had time to have a drink and a rest, would run alongside her to give her motivation, while me and Charlie and a few others would sit there laughing at how seriously they all took it.

Another awkward sports moment was dance. I mean, seriously JFS, you don't offer drama classes but you make us don black Lycra leotards *over* blue Lycra shorts in bodies we are all unsure of, so that we can move around a little bit? That outfit was dreaded and hated by every single one of us. We came in all shapes and sizes and were awkward enough about our changing bodies anyway, and then they went and put us in tight leotards worn OVER, yes, over Lycra shorts. I cringe at the thought even now. We never learned a single dance routine.

In the middle of Year 10, everything changed when I found something that altered my life forever. I began drama classes on a Thursday evening at the Sharon Harris Drama School and I fell in love with drama. Ever since I had done some acting as a child at Crystal Arts, I had always wanted to get more involved in it, and do something that was nothing to do with school. I could be someone completely different in front of the people at Sharon Harris, because they didn't know me and I formed some great friendships. The acting gave me confidence but having friendships with new people who were nothing to do with school really opened up my confidence as I had this whole other social life. And of course, there was a boy.

Sam was one of Sharon's favourite young actors. He'd been with her for a few years and was semi well-known from the work he'd done on TV programmes, commercials and theatre, namely the 'Too Juicy' Fruitella advert. Most of the girls were into him. It was almost as if he was our own mini celebrity over whom we ogled and giggled but would remain almost elusive and totally out of our league and kind of like a fantasy you daydream about, like celebrity crushes tend to be. In my mind, Sam, and others like him, would always be just a fantasy like Jason Donovan had been when I was nine because, well, I was me and they were unattainable.

Sam was so different to the boys at school. He was two years older than me − and when you're sixteen, nearly-eighteen year old boys have way more appeal − and I loved watching him on stage.

At the beginning of each class, we were told what we would be performing that evening, and then we would be split into groups and go off to rehearse. One evening, the gods of teenage crushes were on my side and I was placed in a group with Sam and two other boys − Steve and Jason, who I was already friends with.

I still had quite a skinny frame, thanks to the previous year's near-anorexia, and I wasn't sure if this was attractive or not. I was told more than once by one of the boys in my geography class that my legs were 'disgustingly skinny'. I had not really grown into myself yet and, although I was starting to develop more confidence, I was still painfully self-conscious. Sometimes I thought I looked pretty, and at other times I felt that I was the world's ugliest teenager that ever existed, ever. It didn't help that I was also extremely clumsy.

As Steve, Jason, Sam and I walked towards one of the back

rooms to rehearse, I silently prayed for three things:

1. That I would not trip over my own feet - something I seemed to do quite often;
2. That I would get a part that I would be able to act well in order to impress Sam, who I knew was much more experienced than I was; and
3. That somehow - and I wasn't quite sure how - Sam would decide that he fancied puny, skinny, pale-faced and inexperienced old me.

As we sat down in the small and sparsely furnished room, Sam took control. I was completely shocked, but ecstatic, to learn that he knew my name. We had a lot of fun during that class and our performance was praised by both teachers, probably because Sam was part of the group but, even still, it was an achievement. Other achievements that night, for my part, included the fact that I did not trip over my feet and, on the way out when everyone was saying goodbye, Sam asked me for my phone number.

It was 1999 and not everyone had a mobile phone. Mum got her first mobile when I was about eleven. It was called the Mercury One2One and I used to hold it pretending I was a top female executive, like Elizabeth Perkins in Big or Kelly Lynch in Curly Sue. The phone reminded me of Zack from Saved by the Bell with his huge mobile phone that resembled a cordless home telephone. In 1995, before people spoke on the phone for hours on end, the idiots at Mercury One2One (now TMobile) offered free evening and weekend calls, which they later regretted when they realised how much money they had lost on this service. It worked for me though, as I spent hours in the evening talking on that brick to my friends.

When Sam asked for my number, I had just turned sixteen and for my birthday my parents had given me my first mobile phone. I was so excited to be able to give Sam my mobile number. But at the time it was just natural to give your landline number first. I do miss the days when you waited by your house phone, hoping that the boy would call and you'd scream at your parents every time they tried to use the phone and if they did, and you didn't get a call that night, you'd never know if he tried to call or not. But there was way less confusion than today. Did he text or leave a voicemail or an email or a Facebook message or a Tweet or a comment on Instagram or a message on Whatsapp? No, in those days he either called or he didn't and that was that. Far less complicated. Much more appealing.

That night, when I got home from drama, all I could think about was whether he'd call or text. But of course he didn't. Nor did he call the next day and I decided that he had probably asked for my number as a bet with some of the other boys and I'd now have the awkwardness of facing him the following week. The next day at school I hated boys.

That weekend, I went with a couple of friends to a dance class at Pineapple Dance Studio in Covent Garden. My knees made it hard for me to be flexible enough to dance well and Mum didn't really want me to go, but I convinced myself that I was the same as everyone else and so I would go along to Pineapple and take the class – mainly because anyone who went there was seen as very cool. When I got there, I saw a few Sharon Harris students coming in and out of different classes, ranging from ballet to hip-hop to break-dancing. The fact that my school friends witnessed me greeting people they didn't know made me feel like I wasn't the odd one out for once and I was thrilled that me being there was seen to be a regular occurrence by my drama friends.

Although the class was difficult for me, I was just about able to keep up and I quite enjoyed it. As we walked out, I noticed a voicemail on my mobile. My smile spread from ear to ear as I walked down the steep Pineapple staircase, slow as a snail, listening to Sam's message. People kept pushing past, making tutting sounds as if to say, get out the way. I wasn't really paying attention, I was just focused on the voicemail in which Sam said that he hoped I was having a nice weekend, he really enjoyed working with me on Thursday and I should give him a call if I fancied going out.

I had never been on a date before – apart from when I was thirteen and I had a sort of boyfriend for all of two weeks until he dumped me on the night of his Bar Mitzva – and neither had most of my friends. I discussed the situation in great detail with Charlie before I called Sam back. When he answered the phone, my voice was shaking, but after a few minutes I calmed down and we spoke for about fifteen minutes, which I thought was pretty substantial. He wanted to take me to a bar in Watford called O'Neill's – which, according to my mother, was not a place sixteen year-old Jewish girls went to, but she let me go anyway – and a few of our other friends from drama class were going to come with us.

Mum dropped me off at Harrow station to meet Sam where we would catch the bus to Watford and throughout the whole bus journey, Sam sat next to me with his arm around me. I'd literally never been so happy in all my life. Isn't it funny how, when you're a teenager, feelings and emotions can augment inside you to such an extent that you're just not sure what to do with all the emotion, like it may overflow; it makes you behave like a mad person because everything is just so dramatic! But rewind the clock back and try to remember what it felt like to be a teenager for a minute and you can understand the elation I felt when I had this gorgeous guy whom everyone fancied with his arm around *me*. A number of the other girls from drama class were in the group and I wondered why he'd chosen me out of all of them. As if the emotions of just being with him didn't make me enough of a frenetic mess, at the end of the night he kissed me, and, well, I may as well have spontaneously combusted right on the spot, or later that night when I couldn't sleep because he was all I could think about.

The following Thursday at drama class we were a fully-fledged couple – boyfriend and girlfriend – and I smiled every time Sam referred to me as his girlfriend. It was the first time I ever really felt special.

It didn't take long for me to notice that I liked Sam because of his status within our little 'Sharon Harris bubble'. Had he have been less revered within the company, I don't think he would have had the same appeal, and as I got older, this theme tended to remain the same. Powerful, well-respected or well-known for something or other – that's what did it for me.

I never really got on with Sharon Harris very much. She was the typical 'sweetie dahling' character from Absolutely Fabulous and I was certainly not one of her favourite students. She didn't hesitate to tell you if you had done a bad job and was not afraid to hurt anyone's feelings and I always felt so small around her. She was average height, had strawberry-blonde hair and always wore expensive clothes that suited her just perfectly. Sharon's husband took the money for the classes at the door and I thought that they were the oddest match. He looked more like a builder than the husband of a successful talent agent, but he was a lovely, friendly man and everyone loved him.

Despite my dislike of Sharon and her dislike of me, I loved going to the classes and spent all week looking forward to Thursday nights. I loved drama, adored it. It was, like swimming had been a decade before, *my* thing, just for me and no one else. But Sharon had been right – not that my sixteen year old self would have admitted it. In fact, if my eighteen or even twenty-two year old self had admitted it, I may have been in a very different situation now. However much I loved acting, it didn't come naturally to me. I wasn't the Dakota Fanning or Haley Joel Osment that I would have liked to have been. Had I have met Lee Strasburg in my early years – or any years – and realised the secret weapon behind Method Acting, perhaps I would have done a better job. I had the multitude of feelings and emotions that Method Acting required – I'd certainly been through enough for a sixteen year old – but I was unable to tap into these emotions for some reason and I didn't try hard to tap into them either. I read a script, did the best I could and that was it. I never took it as far as I could have done or should have done. I didn't understand the need to find the depth of the character, to become the character, in the way that I do now and, just like with school, I kind of wish someone would have explained that to me earlier on. I wasn't the natural born actor but when I tapped into it, I was able to find it, and I find it well. But this wasn't school and drama teachers were not expected to find the best in someone who seemed as though they had no talent for it, it wasn't their responsibility like it was with school teachers. It was my responsibility and I let the opportunities pass while I spent all my time and interests on boys and looking good. So, there we go, Sharon, if you're reading this, it turns out you did know what you were doing. But then you already knew that, didn't you.

Despite my lack of natural talent, I landed a few extra parts, a couple of speaking parts (and by that I mean one-liners) and some theatre shows.

One of the first extra roles I got was as a student in Hope and Glory with Lenny Henry. To this day, if I do something to embarrass myself by being inconceivably naïve (it is a recurring theme in my life), my mum labels it as 'a Lenny Henry moment'.

So, we're standing around in our costume uniforms waiting

for the scene to be filmed. It is a scene that will take us from the outside of the school hall, through the doors and into the assembly hall. It was me, about four other girls, and a very tall man. All the others were already inside the assembly hall and I was quite proud that in my first job I was chosen as one of the few who would get the camera right on me as I walked into the assembly hall with a teacher after the assembly had already started. Something had happened to the glidetrack used for the cameras so while they were fixing it we all stayed in our places and had a chat. Whenever we went on these jobs the same three drama schools were represented: Sharon Harris, Bodens and Sylvia Young. We all stayed in our cliques, it was like a competition of whose school was the best, so while hanging around outside waiting for the scene to start, all the stuck-up kids asked each other, and me, who their agent was – it was always the first question. I stayed quiet, and the tall man who was playing the teacher must have thought me to be lonely and said, "Hi, what's your name?" "Lauren," I said. "What's yours?" "Lenny," he replied. I nodded, completely unaware. "So, who's your agent?" I asked, trying to fill the silence, not knowing what to ask so instead following the example of all the other girls. He kind of laughed, then said, "I have a few." "Oh, why? What do you do?" I asked. "I'm a comedian," this tall man called Lenny says. "Oh wow, go on, tell us a joke!" He laughed again, probably at my complete and utter oblivion, and before he had the chance to either tell me that he was Lenny Henry, or tell a joke, the director informed us that the scene would be starting and we should get in our places.

At lunchtime, as we were all sat on steps in our cliques in the playground of this school being used as a film set, Lenny Henry walked past, waved at me, and winked. "Oh my God, did you talk to him??" asked Christina, one of my friends from Sharon Harris. "Err, yeah. We filmed a scene together." I was confused. "You know he's Lenny Henry don't you?!" I'd been told that this show was starring Lenny Henry but I was still stupid enough to miss the fact that it was him, even when he introduced himself as Lenny.

A few weeks later, I received a signed A4 picture of him, with a message on the back. I don't know where that picture is now but the message on the back was taking the mick saying something along the lines of 'tell us a joke'. My mum found it hysterical and I thought it was so sweet of him to find out who my agent was and send me this picture.

I also did other jobs with well-known actors in that time and they were some of the most fun days of my life. I socialised with my Sharon Harris friends on the weekends too. Once, there was an open audition for Hollyoaks (an over-dramatic soap opera featuring heavily-made up, overly tanned girls and the worst actors that ever existed) and although it was an open audition that anyone could attend, Sharon encouraged us to go so we all met up, about twenty of us, and spent the day queuing outside but we were all such good friends by this point that we just had such a laugh.

I was in year 11 at school and we had to start deciding what we wanted to do with the rest of our lives – a tall order for sixteen year olds. I had so many interests, so many things could have been possible with the right guidance (my choices were actress, vet, physiotherapist, interior designer, stay on at sixth form until I knew for sure...) but I chose to go to performing arts school. I was going to be an actress come hell or high water. I was going to get better parts and get famous and earn loads of money to help my parents and be recognised for something other than being the girl with arthritis.

One night I got a call from Steve, sounding rather ominous, saying he needed to tell me something. "Sam isn't who you think he is and me and Jason thought you should know that he's been lying, it's gone on too long." "What do you mean?" I asked. "Lying about what?" It transpired that he was the same age as me, not eighteen – and I'm not quite sure why he had to lie about that because I doubt it would have made a difference – and there were a whole range of other strange things he lied about. Turns out there was a reason for him being such a great actor – he was actually a compulsive liar. He lied about things that seemed so trivial and unimportant that I wondered why he needed to lie about them but I suppose that is what compulsive liars do. I called him and tried to get him to tell me the truth but he just put the phone down.

Jason celebrated his eighteenth birthday on a boat on the Thames and, although Sam and I went there together, I confronted him once we arrived, as I could not wait until the night was over. Being the thespian he was, he caused a scene, of course, and I knew from his reaction that Steve had been right. He had lied to me about his age, his work, his friends, his family – you name it, he lied about it. But I was not going to allow this to ruin my night.

A new boy had started attending drama class a few months previously and he was stunningly beautiful. He had soft blond hair, blue eyes and tanned skin - not features I was used to seeing in my Jewish school. Rob started getting acting work through Sharon almost immediately and he quickly became her new favourite which, again, added appeal. He also happened to be one of the nicest guys I had ever met and we became very friendly.

Before that night on the boat, Rob and I had been speaking on the phone nearly every night, with me complaining that things with Sam weren't great as I didn't trust him, and with Rob listening, subtly trying to convince me that I could do better than Sam. I started to really like Rob but we also managed to build a friendship. The more I got to know him, the more I liked him, and every time I saw him, I had the butterflies that I used to have with Sam but no longer did. I had thought that Sam was the best-looking guy I had ever met, but Rob was something else. He was breathtakingly handsome, but in an unintimidating, 'boy-next-door' sort of way.

Unlike Sam, Rob was interested in the details of my life and, during our hour-long conversations, I would tell him about my experiences with arthritis. He was genuinely interested in my stories and always asked questions. All my school friends knew that I had arthritis and this was something they had always known, so no one ever asked about it. But Rob wanted to know all about it.

Though he asked a lot of questions and listened intently, I don't think Rob really understood what arthritis was or how it affected me, probably because I looked so normal and never showed if I was in pain. Though these were my most stable years, my legs never felt like 'normal' legs; there was always a twinge of pain somewhere, but I tried to ignore it most of the time.

During my argument with Sam on the boat, I told him that it was over and went out onto the deck to find Rob. He was standing there by himself and, as he saw me coming towards him with tears in my eyes, he gave me a hug that made me feel that everything would be OK.

We sat there for hours talking and innocently flirting. Rob put his jacket over me and then decided that since we were actors and were on a boat, we should re-enact the famous scene from the film, Titanic. I stood up on the railing, with Rob behind me with his hands around my waist. My heart was pounding with excitement – until he quoted the words, "do you trust me?" from the movie, and we collapsed with laughter.

We were hysterical for about five minutes until the

laughter started to die off. Then, Rob's hands grasped my waist even tighter, causing my heart rate to speed up in anticipation of what was about to happen. As I turned my head to look at him, he released one hand from my waist, gently placed it on my face and bought me closer towards him as he kissed me. At sixteen years old, it was the most erotic moment of my life and, although we were only young, nothing came close to that moment for me until a very many years later. It was like something out of a film, not just the Titanic part, but the emotions, the utter exquisiteness of the moment. It was perfect.

The cliché of being caught by the ex didn't happen – this wasn't a predictable Rom Com that we were all hoping to be cast in one day – and Sam didn't see us. In fact, Sam went home as soon as our argument ended and I never spoke to him again. He never came back to drama class and none of the others ever heard from him either. I think that he was embarrassed about the fact that everyone knew he had been lying so much.

Although I was very attracted to Rob and enjoyed the time we spent together, and despite our perfect moment on the boat and our undeniable chemistry, I didn't want a relationship with him. I had had a four-month relationship with Sam, which had not turned out the way I thought it would, I was in the middle of my GCSEs and was about to go to Israel for the summer. My head just was not in the right place for another doomed relationship with an actor. Jeez, wasn't I too young to be learning about doomed relationships with actors??

Rob was quite upset at how laid-back I was about the whole situation, as he expected it to go somewhere and considering that I felt as if I had hit the jackpot attracting someone like Rob, I even surprised myself with my reaction. I suppose I was more sensible than I gave myself credit for, or was I? In the end, it turned out to be one of the most stupid decisions I ever made. Had I have made a different choice, I may have been able to avoid the onslaught of heartache that was about to take hold of me the following year.

I kept in touch with him throughout my GCSEs but then I went to Israel for six weeks and everything fizzled after that. We did meet up one more time a few months later, but he told me that it was too painful for him to be around me on our own and not be with me, so he couldn't see me again outside of drama class. It shocked me that he still felt that strongly and I was even more shocked by the fact that I could have that effect on someone. That was not something that I ever thought would happen.

I was upset to lose Rob as a friend and, because I was about to start studying performing arts at college, I wouldn't see him every week as I wouldn't be attending Thursday night drama classes every week, although I still belonged to the agency. I tried to contact him to persuade him to remain friends, but he didn't want to know. I regretted losing him and missed him for a very long time. We also met up one more time around six years later but again, after that one meeting, he didn't want to stay in touch. He is now a successful actor, as I always knew he would be.

Aside from all the teenage crush dramas, I was working hard at school and as we approached our exams at the end of Year 11, I knuckled down to some study in order to pass my GCSEs and couldn't wait to starting Performing Arts School.

Chapter 5

Time to Rebel

I spent six weeks of the summer of 2000 in Israel, staying with my aunt and uncle and two young cousins. I spent a lot of time with cousins and friends I'd grown up with and returned six weeks later, tanned, rejuvenated and ready to start my new life as an adult.

Nanny had taken me shopping to buy me some new outfits for college. I had no idea what one wore for one's first day at college but I wanted to make a good first impression so I settled on black jeans, a black long-sleeve top and a purple PVC jacket (don't worry, this was stylish in 2000 – if PVC was ever considered stylish). Seems strange that I remember what I wore for my first day at college.

A lot of parents pushed their kids to stay on at sixth form and get a good education in the hope they'd go to university and be a lawyer or something equally as generic but Mum really supported my decision in choosing performing arts. I'm not sure if this was because she still believed that I was 'average' and would be unlikely to achieve much if I stayed on at school and had more chance of making it as an actress. She'd given me the lecture on how many actors were out of work compared to those in work but of course, as every actor knows when they first set out, you are totally sure that you will be the 'in work' actor, you are going to make it, end of. So I'm not sure if it was for that reason or if she was just genuinely being supportive and letting me follow my own instincts and find my own path. If I had to choose differently as an adult, I may have done just that, so I think my mum was pretty strong for not getting in the way of 'my dream'.

A friend from school, Nicola, had been intending to study beauty therapy, but she decided at the last minute to try for the same course as me and she got in. At the beginning I had thought that I wanted to do this on my own, as my new challenge, but I became more accustomed to the fact that Nicola would be joining me because when it all began to sink in, I realised that I'd be all alone for the first time ever; the journey to Watford, walking into the class not knowing anyone. It was a slight comfort to have her there in the end.

Most of the students were friendly, but it was a big culture shock to go from such a secluded life in Jewish schools in North West London to a college in Watford with people from every walk of life. One of the girls was nineteen and had a three year-old son, most of the boys were gay or bisexual and most of the girls – all the same age as me – were sexually active. They'd talk about where they had sex with their boyfriends, what form of contraception they used, the positions they tried, and they spoke about it openly, like it was totally normal and me and Nicola would sit there in complete amazement at how little we knew about life. I know that this makes me sound very sheltered, but I had never been exposed to any of this side of life before and it was all new to me. The most sexually active I'd been was when Jonny tried to convince me to give him a blowjob and I got scared and ran off. I *was* sheltered, but I'm not necessarily sure that's a bad thing; we had our childhoods...

So off Nicola and I went, two little Jewish girls from Edgware in our Lois jeans and Buffalo shoes, and rocked up in

Watford and tried to fit in. We didn't necessarily fit in as such, but we soon made friends and integrated with everyone else.

All of a sudden I felt very grown up, and just like that, I felt like I'd outgrown my school friends, most of whom stayed on at sixth form. It was as if I had gone out into the big wide world (albeit only Watford) and they were still none the wiser about what went on outside JFS and all things Jewish and I had no interest in their linear lives where nothing changed or evolved other than their academic achievements. I may have only been in dingy old Watford, but I saw potential for growth, for change, for opportunity and I realised how absolutely insular everything had been up until that point. Danielle went to the college down the road from mine, which she soon dropped out of, and Charlie attended another college where she studied travel and tourism and they were the only ones I stayed in touch with.

Performing Arts was amazing. Why did anyone bother doing anything else? Some classes were a bit boring, so I let my mind wander during these classes; I wandered off to the world of Hollywood and fame and I daydreamed about all the opportunities that were out there. I was so young, I had so much time, anything could have happened and I could have gone anywhere and done anything, especially seeing as I seemed to be all but in remission save the odd pain here or there.

Most of the classes actually weren't boring and we learnt about method acting, Alexander Technique, how to connect with every part of your body and mind in order to access the plethora of emotions that lay inside us and I ate it all up and embraced it all; the humming, the meditation, the pilates, the 'be a tree' or 'find your inner child' moments – every, single pretentious part of it. During breaks from classes we'd take ourselves to the costume department backstage (only the Performing Tarts – as we were known – had access to the costume department), choose an outfit we thought appropriate and wear it for the remainder of the day and I'm not talking dance gear and tutu's, I'm talking bears and Henry VIII and Peter Pan and Ewok. We were 'exploring our creativity', and just being right twats.

The dance teacher, Jane, didn't like me very much, but I had discovered that I could use humour to cover up anything I didn't like about myself and so I became somewhat of a class clown. Although the arthritis hadn't flared for a few years, I still couldn't get my legs into certain positions so, although I tried during the dance classes – and by try I mean I would look at myself attempting tap dancing in the mirror pretending I was Ginger Rogers, having some sort of strange illusion that I actually looked good doing this – I never got very far and succumbed to joking my way through the lessons, which obviously did not go down very well with Jane.

The course was split into three main parts: acting, singing and dancing. The year group was more or less split equally between the three and most of the dancers had been dancers since they were little and to be fair to them, they shouldn't have had people like me in some of their classes, slowing them down. I was an actress and despite the fact that I was certainly not a triple-threat, I loved musicals. I knew I'd never be in one, and that if I was going to follow my dream it would lead me to straight theatre, TV or film, but I just adored musicals. I hadn't yet seen all the musicals I wanted to because I was only sixteen and to see Phantom of the Opera would have cost me my life savings and then some, but I had the soundtracks from nearly all of them. Even though I wasn't a singer per se, our musical theatre classes were my favourite next to the monologue and duologue classes. I really got on with Paul, who took us for musical theatre and I loved every minute of his classes but he ended up getting fired because of his overt interest in sixteen year old girls. However, before I knew this I started taking private singing lessons with him in the hope that I could improve my voice just that little bit more. It wouldn't make me a musical theatre star but any extra talent would increase my chances at finding an agent. Paul gave me a valuable piece of advice: All you need to be a good stage actor is to remember your lines and not bump into things. I was sure there was more to it, but it was a good start. I had the memory thing down, but bumping into things? I had to work on my clumsiness...

For my seventeenth birthday, Mum took me to see Les Miserables and I fell in love with musical theatre and have yet to fall out of love with it. I cried at the end, not because it was sad, but because I was jealous – again – that it wasn't me on stage. This would be a recurring theme in my life any time I visited the theatre or watched the Oscars, Golden Globes, Emmy's, SAG Awards and Grammy's. Yeah, I know what you're thinking. I'm thinking it too.

We took classes on Stanislavski and Method Acting with our teachers Ben and Maz and I got distinctions in every class. I was praised for my monologues, especially the ones where I managed to cry on cue so I suppose I was beginning to tap into the talent a little more but I had a long way to go. I had it all in me, but there was a blockage and unfortunately it would be years until I unblocked it and started releasing my emotions in a way that would enable me to not just have a passion, but be good at it too.

We celebrated the New Year of 2001 and I had been at West Herts College for four months. Nicola, Danielle and I had found new places to go at the weekend. One pub in Stanmore, five minutes from where we lived, was popular with us as all the 'older lot' (as we used to refer to them) hung out there. There were in fact two pubs a few doors down from each other. The first, the Vintry, was very strict about who they let in and, if you weren't over eighteen, you weren't getting through the doors; we were, after all, still sixteen. Every Sunday night we would try to get into the Vintry, fail, and head over to the Crown, as they let everyone in. We never thought to drink alcohol, ironically enough, we just went to socialise and it was basically like being back at JFS with a few other schools thrown into the mix. The Gypsy owned pub was filled with little Jewish school kids. Excellent work.

At the back of the pub was a pool table and we would hang around there, fluttering our eyelashes at the guys playing pool. That is where I met Dave and Mia. Dave was a year older than me and he was going out with Mia. Dave and I clicked straight away, never as anything more than friends, but I felt as if I had known him forever. He introduced me to Mia who, in turn, introduced me to all her friends.

Although Nicola, Danielle and I were the same age, I needed a change. I needed something different to the humdrum banality of my school friends. I wanted to stay friendly with them, but from a distance. So, I began to spend all my time with Mia and her friend, Marina.

Mia and Marina were like no other friends I had had. They were nineteen going on twenty when I was sixteen going on seventeen (and that wasn't intentionally meant to sound like the song out of The Sound of Music) and at the time, this made a lot of difference. They'd done a lot of stuff I hadn't. Marina was originally from Bulgaria and was very tall, with long dark hair and a broad build and had what I can only describe as a very 'eastern European look' about her. Mia was also tall, but naturally very thin. She had no hips and her stomach was completely flat, and she had amazing boobs. I was extremely flat-chested and very envious of Mia's perfect boobs. Blonde hair, flat stomach, big boobs. Hmmm, I wonder why the boys liked her so much...

Dave was the quintessential 'man's man', tall, broad and handsome and looked much older than his seventeen years.

He had just passed his driving test and spent every waking hour in his brand-new maroon Ford Fiesta which at the time was like, *the* best car ever.

Every Thursday, I went with Mia, Marina, Dave and Dave's friends to a club in Watford, called Destiny. Destiny in Watford, it is pretty much as bad as it sounds; slutty girls dressed in tacky clothes, WKD's and Smirnoff Ices and other cheap alcopops for sale, boys roaming around like lions on a hunt, and garage music. Oh but we loved the garage music.

There are not many genres of music that make such a monumental impact on such a lot of people, but still manage to die out before the next generation have had the chance to experience it. By next generation I mean my sister's age. By the time the four years had passed between me starting to go clubbing and Ilana starting to go clubbing, Garage had died and she knew nothing of it. She didn't get how great it was for everyone in a club to all be MCing along to Miss Dynamite's Boo, or Sparks and Kie's Fly Bi – word for word. She would never understand the significance of being on a dance floor when DJ Pied Piper and the Master of Ceremonies were up on stage and called you up to dance on stage with them (if they thought you were fit enough). She'd never get that feeling that only the intense baseline of Garage music can give you, when it travels from the subwoofers through the floor, through your feet and up to your head, causing your face to vibrate and making you feel like you're tripping on acid even if you're not. That genre of music was inspirational in its own way for the tiniest amount of time, but everyone in that time would have been inspired, albeit inspired to do drugs, rob people and bop our heads up and down like pigeons while we held the collars of our denim jackets up so we looked 'bad'.

If I was told that there were auditions being held at Sharon Harris during class on a Thursday evening, I'd pop along to there first, before rushing out the door to get back and get dressed and ready for when Dave would hoot outside my house and I'd go running out, all short PVC skirt, equally tacky top, denim jacket and hoop earrings, promising my parents that I wouldn't be back too late and that everyone dressed like this.

Rob still went to Sharon Harris every week so I'd see him if I went and we'd do the whole civil, 'Hi how are you?' 'Yeah fine thanks and you?' routine and that would be the extent of it.

One of those times when there was an audition, some casting directors had come along to audition for regular sixth formers for Grange Hill and, as any British actor knows, your rep as an actor cannot be substantiated unless you started your career in the BBC studios of Grange Hill.

It turns out, the casting directors liked me and I got a call-back. I went to the second audition which was held in an independent casting suite. "Name, age, agent and profile," said the casting director without even looking at me, as they always do, at which point you're expected to look straight into the camera and say your name, your age, your agent and then turn to each side so they can see your profile and I'd suck in my cheeks and my chin as much as I could. I should have said "Lauren Vaknine, FIFTEEEN, Sharon Harris." It turns out the tight gits at BBC wanted to have actors that looked old enough to play sixth formers – which I did – but were young enough to still be paid under sixteen day rates. So I didn't get the job. Well, I'll never really know if I didn't get it because of that or if I wasn't going to get it anyway but, such is life.

Another example of my near-fame – and this really would have resulted in *actual* fame – was when Sharon sent me to audition for the new Anne Frank film that was being made. I'd just started Performing Arts at West Herts and it would have meant quitting, but that was what we were all there for anyway, wasn't it? Getting famous? Or at least getting acting jobs? So if we got one before, what did it matter? But I was getting ahead of myself.

The audition was held in an old church in Archway and Aba took me, as he often did, come to think of it. He hadn't been around much when I was younger but as the millennium approached, markets weren't what they had been and he kept having to drop more and more days so he was around some days to take me to auditions. He was very proud that I was auditioning for a film about Anne Frank, as I suppose any Jew would be regardless of the fact that Casablanca was nowhere near Amsterdam.

They wanted me to audition for Margot, which I did, by performing my favourite monologue of all time: Lady Jane Grey, A Room in the Tower. The monologue was set in the five minutes before Lady Jane Grey, the poor, condemned Nine Day Queen, was about to be executed and she didn't know if she'd ever see her husband again. I actually performed the monologue quite well, even shedding a tear at the right place, but once again, I didn't take it as far as I should have done with that monologue or any monologue. I didn't even think to look up who Lady Jane Grey was at the time. It didn't occur to me to even attempt to get to know who this character was who was stuck in the Tower of London calling out for someone named Guildford whom at first I thought was a town. How amateur I was. Now when I read that monologue it has a whole new meaning. Anyway, I performed the monologue, and although I criticise my talents now, because of my lack of research and preparation, I couldn't have been as awful as I always seem to think I was. The casting directors sent me out to the waiting room and told me to wait, then came back fifteen minutes later and asked if I'd like to audition for Anne. Does the Pope have a balcony? Yes yes yes! Before I'd even set foot back in the audition room, Aba was on the phone to one of his friends doing his typical Moroccan show-off routine:

"Yes, of course, Lauren's auditioning to play Anne Frank in a HUGE Hollywood movie and of course Lauren will get it because they wanted her for Margot but she was so great that they now want her to play Anne and yes, she will go to Amsterdam to film and we will go with her, of course, me and Marsha, and we will be parents of a famous child." Seriously, that is what he does all the time, bless him.

So I auditioned for Anne. Not once, not twice, not even three times. They called me back on four separate occasions until Aba's car practically drove *itself* to Archway and they'd narrowed down the part of Anne Frank between me and this one other girl, Hannah something.

In the end, as is sod's law, the other girl got it. They stood in front of the two of us, giving us the respect we deserved after such a grueling auditioning process and said that at this point it really was not about the acting as we were both equally as good (really?!) and it really just came down to who looked more the part. I was quite pale, perhaps a little too olive, but I was skinny and had dark hair and dark black circles under my eyes which in my opinion was basically the epitome of Anne Frank. (In retrospect, perhaps I should have laid off the vanity and concealer for a few weeks.) It was kind of annoying because if I would have stayed as Margot, maybe I would have still been in the film but they said I looked too young and not frumpy enough to play Margot. I took that as a compliment.

I was pissed off. It was my first real major chance at anything big. It wasn't a one liner every few episodes in Grange Hill, or a dog food commercial, it was a real film in which Sir Ben Kingsley would have played my father! It took me ages to get over the fact I didn't get it. Two things led me to resent losing out on that part for a longer time than was appropriate: Sharon decided to literally not talk to me again. It just wasn't good enough that I didn't get it, even though I proved myself by getting so far into the audition process. That was basically the end of me at Sharon Harris. The second thing happened about eight years later when my mum showed me an article that she should not have shown me: Britain's Under 25's Rich List. And who was on it? None other than the girl I lost out on the part of Anne to. In the bit that said, 'why is she so rich?' it genuinely said, 'because she played Anne Frank in Anne Frank: The Whole Story'.

So that was that. Back to college and agentless. I just figured I'd stay in college for the two years, then go to uni to study drama or to drama school if I could get a bursary or get an agent straight out of college. Simples. Looking back on what happened not so long after that failed audition, I reckon many bad things would not have happened had I have got that part but I'm not one for shoulda woulda couldas. Oh, and to this day I still adore that Jane Grey monologue.

Back to college life: Mia often picked me up from college saving me from having to get the sodding bus which took forty-five minutes on what should have been a fifteen minute journey. Mia had two other friends, one of whom was Lana. She was one of those people whom others find hard to approach, you know, the bitchy looking, unapproachable type. She was tall with long, dark, shiny hair, perfectly-sculpted high cheekbones and piercing green eyes. Sometimes, if she was not smiling, it would seem as if she were throwing evil looks at me. She was stubborn and argumentative and really, quite rude most of the time. Lana didn't like me very much at the beginning and I never really understood why, but it didn't bother me as she rarely went out with us. She was in a serious relationship and hated clubbing, dancing, drinking and generally having fun and, on the occasions that she did come out, she would spend the whole evening texting her boyfriend. I didn't bother to make much effort with her, as she was always quite rude and that's how things were between us for a while.

Zoe was also hard to approach if you didn't know her, but she and I clicked instantly. I met her in Mia's garden when we were celebrating her twentieth birthday with a barbeque. I thought that she was Mia's age, if not older. She had a worldly and mature air about her and I was amazed to find out that she was the same age as me. Zoe also had a serious boyfriend (was I the only single one?) but she loved going out with all of us.

At college, we were about to start casting for our pre-Easter musical, A Chorus Line. We watched the film, learned the songs and read the script so that we would know which parts we would audition for.

But... why can't things get shittier when they're already shitty? Why do things go from amazing to unimaginably deplorable in the time that it takes you to say Juvenile Rheumatoid Arthritis? Just as I decided to really go for it and audition for a lead part after the Anne Frank situation had given me the confidence, my knees accumulated ridiculous amounts of fluid and swelled almost overnight.

I was shocked. This hadn't happened for years and in that time I had grown from child to (nearly) adult. I was still attending two-monthly appointments for my eyes at St. Thomas' Hospital and had been transferred over to Middlesex Hospital, also in central London, for my joints as I was now too old for Great Ormond Street. These appointments were sporadic, every six months maybe, and I usually came away feeling happy with myself. But now, I didn't understand what was going on. The last time my knees had been like that I'd been a child. I was now an adult so everything seemed different, somehow out of context. My knees were so swollen that for the second time in my life, I had to have them drained without a sedative.

Mum was with me but I knew what was coming so I just

panicked as I lay on the bed waiting for the numbing cream to settle in. After what seemed like a lifetime, out came Dr. Smith with her huge needle and frosty disposition and she began the procedure. When she injected the left knee it felt as if the needle had hit a bone deep in the knee and it hurt in a different way to the last injection – a more muscular pain.

Not too much attention was paid to the fact that I thought something had really hurt me, as if the needle had hit a spot it shouldn't have. I was told that that I was being silly: "Lauren, if you could deal with this when you were a child, you can deal with it now." Dr. Smith, delightful as always. I knew my own body, though, and something just didn't feel right.

Ever since then, in the soft part of my knee next to the kneecap where the steroid was injected, I have a very deep dent. A few days after a knee-draining, the knee should be exercised to build up the muscles around the joint. I was in so much pain for so long that I could barely move my knee. The muscle started wasting away and, in its place, I was left with a deep dent and a constant reminder of that particular injection.

Not even a couple of months before, I was auditioning for Anne Frank and Grange Hill, I belonged to a reputable drama agency, I was doing well at college and had a great social life but all that changed with the click of a finger and the insertion of a needle.

I went back to college on crutches a few weeks later and still auditioned for the musical, but I did myself so much damage practicing the dance that would have been my audition piece that by the time I had the audition, I couldn't put down the crutches and do the dance. I was given a part, but not a very big one, and I was devastated.

The flare kept getting worse. My knees and ankles were stiff, swollen and very sore. I was on crutches most of the time and I was angry. I was just starting my life as an adult and everything had been going so well, I was excited for life. I had new friends, a new career path and I was healthy. Up until that point.

When I was younger, the arthritis and uveitis would never flare at the same time, but now, as well as the flare in the knees and ankles, my eye became significantly more misty and blurry.

On going to see Dr. Graham at St Thomas', we were told that after fourteen years of daily steroid eye drops and a lot of inflammation, a cataract had started to grow. It was at the early stages, but was likely to grow more quickly than most cataracts due to the circumstances and this was why my eye was so misty, it was the cataract not the cells. I was told that the eye drops would not be able to control it, but the inflammation was getting worse as the cataract developed and this was not helping the situation.

It was not a simple matter of removing the cataract as with normal cases. The greater the inflammation, the more dangerous it would be to tamper with the eye. The pressure in my eye was also dropping rapidly, with my right eye measuring around 5 or 6 when normal eye pressure should be 12 or 13. As it was too dangerous to remove the cataract, the next step was to get the inflammation down so that removing the cataract would be an option. I was given new drops on top of my usual ones and was now taking an average of twelve drops per day into the eye. This still didn't work and my vision was becoming worse by the day.

The summer soon arrived and I was determined not to let my recent misfortune affect my new-found independence. Danielle, Nicola, Charlie and I had booked our first girls' holiday to Tenerife. Everyone we knew was going, including Gemma and all her friends. I was a bit worried about whether I would cope for two weeks away from my family if I was in pain. I knew that if things were difficult for me, my friends wouldn't understand, they were seventeen year old girls without a care in the world. But I didn't want my first proper holiday away from family to be tainted by those thoughts. I wanted to be the normal seventeen year old who has her first holiday with her friends and sees it as a rite of passage, not something to dread.

We felt we had outgrown The Crown – and by we I mean the whole of North West London under twenty-two – and we found a new pub in which to congregate and not drink alcohol. It was called the Abercorn. It was packed almost all the time, but especially so on Sunday nights. About 90% of the patrons were young, Jewish non-drinkers. They could not have taken very much money, but our whole crowd was there and we began looking forward to our evenings at the Abercorn as much as we looked forward to going clubbing. The summer was the best time at the Abercorn also, because we'd all sit outside.

One night we were sitting around a table in the beer garden and I got talking to Edgware's resident 'bad boy', Michael. All I had ever heard about this guy was bad. When I was still at JFS and got the train into Edgware station, where he and his crew used to hang around all day, every day, I saw him push an elderly man to the floor. I never forgot that sight or the sound of the man falling. I have two weaknesses in life: animals and elderly people. I am the person who stops and asks random elderly people at the bus stop if they want a lift home (they always say no because they're scared), or ask if I can help them with their shopping bags, and I always call the RSPCA if I suspect animal cruelty. These are the two things I cannot stomach and I remember so clearly him pushing this old man down then walking away nonchalantly. I remembered seeing him a hundred times at Edgware station, but I'd never spoken to him. He was known for beating people up for no reason, he took and sold drugs and was generally not a very nice person, but he was in our crowd with the other boys that my friends had grown up with and for some reason I pushed the memory of the old man – and the warning signs – to the back of my mind because I needed something to distract me. I was intrigued by Michael. He was by no means good-looking, being short and skinny with curly brown hair and evil dark eyes, and wasn't even particularly nice, but I was drawn in by the excitement of danger and after that evening at the pub, we started talking a lot more and we fell into a pattern of the entire crowd of us going to Destiny on a Thursday together, and to The Abercorn on a Sunday together. We were like one big, warped, fucked-up family.

Michael had been thrown out of home at a young age and lived in a small bungalow near my house. I spent nearly all my free time, including time when I was supposed to be at college, with him. Nothing happened for a while, we were just friends and I loved being surrounded by the adventure and spontaneity of it all. His lackeys would turn up at his house to give him money all throughout the day and night and his two phones never seemed to stop ringing. Everyone seemed to be scared of him, but I liked the fact that whenever I turned up at the pub with him, people were shocked and were talking about us and we garnered some sort of warped respect.

Michael didn't really know much about my illness, and I worked hard to keep it that way. I didn't think he'd be interested if he knew and I wanted him to see me as someone different to who I really was. I was painfully embarrassed about my arthritis.

Before I left for Tenerife, we welcomed a new addition to our group. We had met Nicole in Destiny one night, the conversation revolving around a guy that both her and Mia had been out with. Nicole became as much a part of our group as the rest of us and she really balanced us out by being the least confrontational and argumentative out of all of us. She was like the mother hen of the group. The five of us – and sometimes Lana – would walk into Destiny with our bad boys every Thursday, thinking we were untouchable. Everyone found us intimidating and we became known as 'The Scorpions', but we reveled in it.

Part of me was turning into this 'scorpion', and the other part of me was still so naïve, believing all the excuses and reasons Michael had for things I found strange and questioned.

In between meeting Michael (at the point when we were still just friends who saw each other at the Abercorn and Destiny and spoke on the phone) and going to Tenerife, I met Lee. He was introduced to me by a friend from college and was what parents would refer to as a 'nice boy' and we got into a relationship. It was as if my college life and social life were two separate entities. At this point, Michael and I were just friends and I didn't know if it would develop into anything. A part of me wanted to see if this would make Michael jealous and we drifted during the three months I was with Lee.

With Lee, there wasn't the same excitement that I had felt when I met Sam, or the way my tummy tied in knots and my heart pounded whenever I was around Rob, and he certainly didn't offer the same dangerous thrills that Michael did, but he treated me wonderfully and my parents loved him. I ended up losing my virginity to him, and I was fine with that, I was seventeen and a half and in a relationship with a guy who cared about me, but he was not what I was looking for at that time and while I was in Tenerife, I cheated on him with one of Gemma's friends. With the community we came from being so small, Lee quickly found out about my antics in Tenerife before I even got back, but I brushed it aside and didn't really care. I didn't once consider his feelings. I had stopped considering anyone's feelings.

Nicole also came to Tenerife with some other people, but ended up spending most of her time with me. We called Mia every day and I couldn't wait to get back to see Michael, as he had also been on holiday for two weeks.

We got back from Tenerife on the Thursday and that Sunday, we all went to the pub. I hadn't expected Michael to be back but, to my surprise, he walked into the pub, straight up to me and I was surprised at how happy I was. It turned out that he had been deported from Ayia Napa for selling drugs – or something along those lines – but I didn't care. Before I knew it, we were in a relationship.

My girlfriends were slightly worried, as they knew him very well and were aware of his reputation, but they let me get on with it all the same. It was part of our lives and we were all as bad as each other.

Nicole was studying beauty therapy at a college near me, but we weren't interested in college. She would pick me up in the middle of the day and we would go to Michael's house to sit and smoke weed with him. This is when I found out that marijuana could relieve pain and as I didn't want to be slowed down by the arthritis at a time when my life was moving at such a fast pace, I started to smoke it nearly all the time. It completely relaxed my whole body to the point where I couldn't feel the pain any more. Michael was dealing, so we didn't have to pay for it and soon I was smoking an eighth of skunk a day. I didn't even smoke hash, which is weaker, I went from being a T-totaller to smoking an eighth of the strongest stuff there is every single day. Although Nicole did partake in the occasional joint smoking session, I don't think she was happy with the amount I was smoking on a daily basis.

My parents were becoming increasingly worried about me and all we did was argue. I couldn't bear the fact that they were trying to stop me doing the things I wanted to do, even though any parent would have done the same. I made excuses for Michael and tried to portray him as some sort of saint, but they had heard about him and knew who he was. They tried to stop me seeing him, but it didn't work. I was angry at the world and became angrier by the day, wondering what the point would have been of trying at college, or being a 'good girl', when ultimately, the arthritis would find a way to ruin stuff. I would start fights in Destiny with anyone, just for looking at me and knowing that my girls were standing behind me made me feel invincible, albeit very stoned.

I think I knew that at some point soon, my life was going to come to a halt again because of the arthritis, after so many years of thinking it might be over. I can't even articulate the anger that I felt towards this realisation. You grow up with an illness, it changes your childhood but then, you become a teenager and it goes away. You're more appreciative and grateful than most people would be because you know the difference, you remember what life was like with the illness and you can appreciate and recognise how good life is without it. You plan a life. You let yourself be happy and excited. But God has other plans and just like that your world changes. My only way of dealing with this was by rebelling against everything I had ever known.

On more than one occasion, I had such big screaming matches with Mum that she grabbed my clothes out of the wardrobe, threw them in a black bin bag and told me that if I wanted to be with him and act like he acted, then I could go and live with him and get the hell out of her house. Twice, I actually took the bags, and anything else I could grab at the time and left. I would walk round to Mia's house – black sack in one hand, cigarette in the other, and moan about how awful my mother was.

One night when this happened, Mia and I drove down to Hemel Hempstead to meet some of the boys who were looking for people who owed them money to beat them up. I would have been unrecognisable to anyone who had known me before and, of course, Michael never tried to do anything to ease the situation because he wasn't about that. He didn't care what my parents thought, or anyone else for that matter.

After a while, and quite predictably, things with Michael weren't as much fun as they had been at the beginning. He already 'had' me, so he didn't have to try anymore and he knew that because I was sucked in by the whole situation, it really didn't matter how he treated me. He spoke about me with a lack of respect in front of other people and made me feel awful about myself by telling me that I was fat and ugly, that I had a 'weird' body and that no one would find me attractive.

In spite of this, he managed to get me to sleep with him. It was awful. I only agreed to do it because he accused me of being a little girl who never wanted to do anything else except kiss, watch movies and smoke weed. He also told me that if I didn't sleep with him, he would break up with me. I was seventeen and didn't want to feel like a little girl, so I gave in. I never enjoyed it, especially because he'd be rude about it afterwards, but I felt as though it was out of my hands.

It continued like this for a while and I often thought about Rob and how things would have been if I were with him right now, instead of Michael. I knew I would be a great deal happier and he would probably make me feel better about my health situation, and yet I could not bring myself to leave Michael. I couldn't understand why – I wasn't even attracted to him. I was, however, infatuated with him. I wanted to be able to get up one day and tell him that it was over, but I just couldn't bring myself to do it and, as time went on, things got worse and worse.

One evening, Michael and I were sitting on the couch watching Eastenders and, after his usual verbal attack about how vile I was, he told me to go into the bedroom. That night, I decided to stand up for myself and tell him that I did not want to have sex with him. With no warning, he threw me from the sofa onto the floor, pinned my hands down with his left hand, ripped off my trousers and climbed on top of me. I struggled, but to no avail - he was too strong. I shouted at him to get off me and then tried to scream when I realised he was not listening, but he slapped his hand over my mouth, hitting my lip against my tooth and making it bleed. His hand was over my mouth the whole time and I could barely breathe, as my mouth was filling up with blood and my nose was blocked from crying.

I lay there, helpless, looking up at the cracked ceiling with tear-filled eyes. I remember so vividly the mixture of smells - his Emporio Armani aftershave and the stench of weed that clung to every part of the house. I could taste the rusty flavour of the blood filling my mouth and felt beads of sweat falling from his face onto mine, as my hips were battered by the thrusting and my back burned by the carpet underneath me. As he had one hand holding my arms and the other over my mouth, he had nothing to support him, so all his weight was resting on his hands, which gripped onto me with strength that I never realised he had. The bones in my hands and arms felt as if they were being crushed and rubbed vigorously against the hard carpet. Before ever talking about this, when trying to remember what had happened and start working through it, all I could remember was a pink broom. I think at some point during the ordeal I'd given up and I tilted my head backwards and all I could see was a pink broom standing in the corner of the kitchenette. That broom stands out in my memory more than anything from those few monstrous minutes.

It happened very quickly, over before my brain could even register what had happened. When he had finished, he spat on my face, removed himself and spoke only to tell me how disgusting I was for coughing in his face. I got up, bruised, bleeding and humiliated, pulled on my tracksuit bottoms and, without saying a single word, I left the house and walked to Mia's.

I couldn't even talk. I had no words, just tears streaming silently down my face, as I walked alone down the dark street. I felt empty but, in spite of the numbness, the tears kept coming. I bought a bottle of water from the off licence in Glengall Road, swirled some around my mouth and spat it out in the road to get rid of the blood. I poured it over my hands to wash the grazes caused by the carpet, wiped them dry on my ripped trousers, lit a cigarette, and carried on walking.

I never told Mia what had happened. I just said that Michael and I had had an argument, which is why I was crying, and I didn't want to go home just yet. She didn't seem too worried and didn't question how I looked. Eventually, I did walk home, in the pouring rain. I didn't know what else to do apart from sit on the grass outside my house, with the rain pouring down on me, in the hope that the rain would wash away what had just happened. I wanted it to cleanse me. I wanted it to get rid of this feeling that I feared would never, ever leave me. I wanted to be my old, innocent self. I just wanted to turn back the clock more than anything I'd ever wanted to do.

The rain didn't cleanse me or make me feel any better. In fact, I felt more than exploited, I felt dirty and used and I also believed that it was probably my own fault for putting myself in such close proximity with a guy like Michael, just because I was excited by the danger. I just hadn't realised that the danger would involve me. How much more stupid could I have been? I made this happen myself, I thought. I didn't know how to deal with it, so I chose the easy option and didn't deal with it. The night that it happened was the last night I cried about it, and the last night that I even thought about it.

Eight years passed before I told anyone what happened. I made myself believe that it never happened. I worked out that this self-delusion would be easier to deal with than the feelings I was experiencing at that moment.

Somehow, I tricked my brain into believing what I wanted to believe and I never admitted it to myself or anyone else. Only recently have I started talking about the experience and dealing with it, which has been very hard, but it has also made me realise that, if I had dealt with it at the time, I may not have had to endure the ill health that followed. Emotional baggage is far more dangerous than we imagine.

I was at least wise enough to make the decision to end the relationship after that ordeal, but the anger I had felt before it now turned into pure rage. I was also angry that, from now on, I would have to pay for my weed.

After that night, all my energies were directed into thinking about Michael. I seemed to have forgotten what he had put me through – my brain had literally blocked it out. For some reason, I was pining over him, which makes absolutely no sense to me now. A few weeks later I tried to speak to him but he didn't want to know. Maybe he knew that what he had done was wrong and didn't know what to say, or perhaps he was just evil and heartless. Knowing what I know now, I suspect the latter. As he wouldn't speak to me, there was only one thing I could do and that was to seek revenge.

Michael had a lot of enemies, but there was one in particular who he really hated. I met Jake through Tarek, who I had recently become very friendly with. Jake and Michael had fallen out over a girl. Michael always wanted her but she always wanted Jake and they were together for a long time but it was common knowledge that they'd recently split.

Tarek came to pick me up from college one afternoon and Jake was in the car with him. Jake was mixed-race with light skin and dark hair, and he was tall, handsome and charismatic – quite different from Michael. I was instantly attracted to him and, as I sat in the passenger seat of Tarek's car, singing along to Tupac's rap song 'Hit 'em, Up', Jake leaned over from the back seat and started rapping the lyrics with me. When the song finished, he asked me how I knew the lyrics to a gangster rap song (it did look quite out of the ordinary and always seemed to take people by surprise). I told him how much I had always loved Tupac and how upset I was when he was killed. I particularly loved the lyrics to his songs and had a book of poems that he had written, entitled 'The Rose That Grew from Concrete'. I offered to show it to Jake, as the poems portrayed a side to Tupac that most people didn't know. Jake told me that he felt a strong connection to Tupac and knew that he would die early, just like Tupac did, "I'll be lucky if I make it to my twenty-first birthday," he said nonchalantly. I didn't pay too much attention at the time.

Apart from the fact that I was very attracted to Jake – physically, but most of all, intellectually, and on some sort of spiritual level – I also knew that it would destroy Michael's ego if he discovered that anything was happening between Jake and me. Jake took my number and we started texting each other day and night.

He was originally from Derby but his family were pretty messed up so he came to London to live with his grandma when he was a young teenager. His grandma lived round the corner from Maytree Close, and we knew her well. She had a really strong Jamaican accent and despite her slight frame, she always had huge, strong dogs that seemed to drag her as she walked. Jake had moved out of his grandma's and he was living in a room in a shared flat above a shop that had three bedrooms and one bathroom that was shared between him, Paul and two Polish girls living in the third room and I spent a great deal of time there with him and his best friend, Paul. Nicole and Mia would sometimes join us.

Jake had somewhat of a menagerie going on in his tiny room. Despite the tight space, he had a snake, two hamsters and a cat. Not a small, sorry-excuse for a snake, but a huge, fully grown python called Daks that lived in a tank that was about as big as his bed. I had always had a fascination with snakes but was scared of this one and I hated watching Jake feed Daks dead mice. The cat, Pepsi, was always out and about and most times, if you were driving past the front of the shop, you could see her sitting on the window frame outside the room. The room stank something rotten, what with all those animals and Jake used to spray toilet spray in his bedroom because he couldn't afford candles and ever since then the smell of toilet spray makes me gag.

To complete the working-class, delinquent version of Siegfried and Roy's fantastical menagerie, Paul had a tortoise, which I later adopted when he went into prison and had no one to look after him. I named him Tupac ShaTortoise. When it came down to it, Jake and Paul were both petty criminals, kids who had come from nothing and had to do what they could to survive, but under it all, they were good people and Jake had some serious intelligence hidden away under all the adversity. Plus, I have a lot of time for anyone who likes animals.

Jake told me all about Natalie and the reason behind their break up. She was pregnant and they were planning on keeping the baby but things were bad between them so she ended up having an abortion and that was that.

Gemma's eighteenth birthday was around the corner and, although Gemma was not in the same crowd as me (she was sensible), she was still a very good friend so, even though I really wasn't in the mood, I agreed to go to Destiny to celebrate her birthday.

Just over a week before Gemma's birthday, after staying at college for the entire day (unusual for me), I went shopping with Mia to the Broadwalk, a small shopping centre in Edgware. I had nothing to buy, but didn't want to go home and, as there was nothing else to do, we mooched around there for a while. As we approached Lindy's – an open-plan café in the middle of the Broadwalk – we saw crowds of people clustering around the TV on the café wall.

We couldn't see very well because of the crowds, but what we could see was that it was showing some apocalyptic CNN news footage.

Soon afterwards, Mum phoned me on my mobile urging me to come home immediately, as terrorists had hijacked planes and flown them into the Twin Towers of the World Trade Center in New York and she was sure that something was about to happen in London.

What had just happened was huge – in fact, it changed history. The whole world stood still on the 11th September 2001. I did go home shortly after, but not before I had argued with my mother and told her that she was stupid for thinking that just because it had happened in the States, it would happen here too. Being the miserable person that I was at the time, I just felt the need to cause an argument.

The day of Gemma's birthday, exactly one week after the tragedy in New York, I began to suffer from an awful stomach ache, unlike anything I had had before. Nicole and I were at my house and she suggested that I smoke some more weed to smother the pain, but that didn't work. I could barely move. I went to the toilet and out of nowhere poured abnormal amounts of blood.

I couldn't understand it, because it wasn't the time for my period. Jake took me to the doctor, along with Nicole. I went in on my own and suggested that Jake and Nicole stay at Jake's friend Damon's house opposite the surgery.

The doctor asked me if there was a chance that I could be having a miscarriage. A feeling of despair washed over me as I denied it, knowing that this was exactly what it was. When she asked me about my sexual activity, I told her that while having sex the condom had split. I was too embarrassed to tell the truth, and a part of me still didn't really believe it. She checked me over and confirmed that I was having a miscarriage and was about seven weeks along in the pregnancy but, as this was only the beginning of the miscarriage, I should go to a family planning clinic as soon as possible. When I climbed back into Jake's car, I answered his and Nicole's concerned questions with a flippant, "I dunno really, she thinks I might be having a miscarriage." Although I tried to make them believe that I didn't agree and didn't need to go to the clinic, Jake drove me there anyway, saying that if I was having a miscarriage, it should be dealt with properly. His genuine concern for my wellbeing made me feel a bit emotional. I got out of the car with Nicole and pretended to go into the clinic, but we didn't actually go.

For some reason I didn't want to. I knew what was happening and would deal with it myself. Luckily, I had been a bit more cautious with Jake, so I knew it was due to Michael and the dates added up and that disgusted me. I managed to convince myself that it had happened because a condom had split.

Nicole was worried and stood by the entrance to the clinic with me and urged me to go in but said she'd support me if I really didn't want to. We waited there for ten minutes then went back to the car and just told Jake that everything was OK.

Jake and Damon drove us to Gemma's party at Destiny and said that they would pick us up later. I couldn't enjoy myself. The pain had started again but, this time, it was really bad and getting worse by the second. Dragging Nicole with me, I rushed to the toilets in the club and there, in Destiny's toilets, what I assume was the zenith of the miscarriage, left my body. That feeling is indescribable. What looked like clumpy pieces of clotted blood and liver fell into the toilet and I felt sick to the stomach. I didn't know when it would end or how I would know when it was over. Would it stop and then start again later, perhaps in the club itself or outside on the street? I didn't have a clue. The hardest thought to accept was that those 'clumps of liver' were in fact a baby. This was the most difficult realisation that my mind has ever had to come to terms with.

I cannot recall how long I was in that toilet or when I left. I really do not remember my feelings and emotions during those few hours of my life. Jake and Damon came to pick us up quite soon afterwards and I didn't mention it. I couldn't. Nicole was the only person who knew. Even though I hadn't known that I was pregnant, I still felt a tremendous sense of loss. The baby was gone – the physical remnants of what Michael had put me through were there no more but, as the days went by, my emotional pain got worse and worse.

There were two people who I wanted to tell, but I couldn't tell either of them. I wanted to tell Mum so that she could give me a hug and tell me that everything would be OK, but I knew I couldn't do that to her; she would be distraught. I also wanted to tell Michael. Even though it was his fault that I was going through this, I felt as if I needed him, so I called him. Big mistake.

He accused me of lying, told me that it had never happened and that I was making it all up to get attention. He said that if it had happened, it was probably Jake's baby. He knew the truth, but he was too selfish to admit it or to help me and so he did what he did best and screamed and swore at me until I put the phone down.

The whole ordeal had affected me so badly that I developed insomnia – and this in spite of the copious amounts of weed I was smoking. I was hurting from what Michael had done to me and what had happened because of it; I was hurting because he wasn't talking to me and that I couldn't talk to my mum. I felt so lost. Dave would bring me more weed whenever he could, but it wasn't helping any more. My joints were getting worse by the day and my emotional pain was unbearable. I was slowly sinking into a deep and powerful depression, but I never realised it at the time and so, as with everything else, I never faced it. I would sit in my room or alone at college just reading through the poems in Tupac's poem book, The Rose That Grew From Concrete, underlining all the bits I felt were relevant to me.

Jake, however lovely he was, was by no means straight-laced. He didn't work so he had to find other ways to make money. Naturally, I participated in all of his illegal and immoral endeavours. One of these 'ventures' was selling weed, something that I didn't think was so terrible at the time. Everyone I knew smoked it, and we had to get it from somewhere, so it might as well be from Jake. I made all the phone calls, weighed up the packets and accompanied Jake to drop them off to our friends.

Another way Jake made money was credit card fraud. During this period of my life, I felt as though I was not really me. It was as if I was watching myself from above. I could see all the things I was doing and how I was acting and the old me knew it was all completely wrong, but it didn't matter, I couldn't escape from the new Lauren because, the more hurt I caused, the less I would hurt. This was of course complete and utter nonsense, but every day I sank further and further into depression and so the rebellion made sense in my head. Every day, I would eat less than the day before and sleep less than the previous night. I had no concept of day and night, right and wrong. A minute didn't go by when I didn't think about Michael and I started obsessing over the baby that I had miscarried, which made no sense as I hadn't known that I was pregnant until I lost it. The only way I could cope with it all was to keep myself drugged up and busy doing anything and everything that would get Michael's attention.

Drug dealing and credit card fraud were on the top of that list. Jake would make me dress in nice clothes so that I looked classy and trustworthy and we would buy items in local shops with credit cards that Jake had stolen from the postman. I bought car stereos and amps, mobile phones, televisions, jewellery and Playstations and, as we bought each item, we would find someone from Jake's crowd to sell them to.

As a thank you, Jake decided to teach me how to drive. Ironically, the first car park he ever took me to was Stanmore Orthopaedic Hospital, where I had been diagnosed sixteen years earlier. We swapped seats and he told me what to do. Shock horror, I was stoned, and drove the car straight into a tree. I apologised profusely, but Jake wasn't bothered at all, saying that it didn't matter because the car only cost £70 from the breakers' yard.

I was selling drugs and doing credit card fraud, while selling the illegal goods to other drug dealers and driving around with a man who was constantly stoned and had no driver's license, in a £70 car with no insurance. You can only imagine how vile I must have been to my parents at the time.

Jake and Michael had many mutual friends, which was strange considering how much they hated each other. One evening, while I sat waiting for Jake to put petrol in the car at Elstree Hill petrol station, I noticed Michael's car pulling up right beside us. My heart pounded. Michael obviously hadn't realised who we were, otherwise I doubt that he would have chosen that particular petrol pump. As Jake got back in the car after he'd paid for his petrol, he looked over to the car on the left and, being the cheeky chappie that he was, rolled down the windows.

Three of their mutual friends were in the car with Michael and they exchanged hellos. I didn't know what to do or where to look, but I managed to look calm and collected as I tried to show that I was with Jake and Michael was single and on his own. Michael became understandably aggravated and got out of the car, slammed the door and walked into the petrol station shop. His anger wasn't under control at the best of times due to his crazy split personality, a dysfunctional upbringing and a generous daily helping of cocaine. This chance meeting wasn't helping and it was followed by a typical show of 'manliness' – a car race. Both cars pulled out of the petrol station at the same time and roared up the road. I clutched my seat as Jake overtook Michael at 90 miles an hour on a residential road with only one lane. Jake looked at Michael and laughed in his face as we overtook him and sped off. Michael's passengers were laughing hysterically, which must have got to him even more and, as we passed him, I saw the rage on his face as his veins protruded from his forehead.

The next day we went to visit Jake's dodgy friend, Connor, at the breakers' yard and traded in the old car for a different one. Connor was one of the scariest looking human beings I've ever met in my entire life. I could barely look at him let alone talk to him.

A few weeks later, Jake started acting very strangely with me. One lunchtime, when Nicole and I had gone to meet Jake and Damon in a pub called The Leather Bottle in Stanmore, Nicole and I waited until Jake had gone to the bar and then checked his phone. We found loads of messages from Natalie on there and, although I didn't have time to read them before he came back, I knew those messages had been from that week. My heart sank as I knew what was about to follow. Sure enough, a few days later, Jake told me that he didn't want to be with me anymore as he and Natalie had got back together. Soon afterwards, I found out that this was because she was pregnant again and, as the baby was his, he was doing the honourable thing. But, as usually happens in these situations, they soon broke up again after they decided not to keep the baby, again.

I was distressed by this break-up, mainly because it meant I would now be alone with no distraction from my nightmarish thoughts of Michael. As crooked as Jake was, he never once disrespected me and always made me feel nice about myself. This I knew I would miss once I fell back into the hole of my depression, fuelled by thoughts of Michael and all that went with it.

One silver lining was that Mia and Zoe had broken up with their boyfriends and so we could all be heartbroken together. To try to fix our broken, teenage hearts, we went out nearly every night of the week and, one night, in Destiny, I saw Natalie. She was probably one of the most intimidating people I had ever come across, even though she was tiny. What made matters worse was that every time I was anywhere she was going to be, and she heard that I was there, she would tell people that if I came in she'd beat me up for going out with Jake. All those times I'd run away and not face her but this time, I put on my 'hard' face and walked in straight past her, letting her know just with my confidence that she couldn't and hadn't beaten me. At first she said nothing and just looked on, but then Mia introduced us and before I knew it, we were chatting like old friends. She took my number and soon became the seventh addition to our group.

What I had never realised was that she was just like us. She had been going out with Jake on and off for three years and was in love with him, so it was no wonder that she had hated me. I had only been thinking about myself when I went out with him and had not understood why she felt as she had.

Natalie and I shared the same pain. She had had an abortion and I had had a miscarriage. I felt that this made us sound cheap and hated the fact that this was how I labelled myself. We never spoke about it to anyone but each other, and it was a comfort to know that there was someone who really understood how I felt.

From that moment, Natalie and I were inseparable. She was unemployed at the time and, when I wasn't at college, we drove around together, sometimes accompanied by Nicole, discussing our problems and smoking weed.

In spite of this friendship with Natalie, I still couldn't change the way I was feeling. The miscarriage had really affected me and I started to realise what it actually meant and what had happened. I felt that I needed closure with Michael and could not move on with my life properly. I was smoking myself into oblivion to stop the pain in my knees, could do nothing about my ever-decreasing vision and felt trapped in my own life.

My legs were in so much pain while I was clubbing that I wanted to cry. It wasn't an option for me to go home and rest, as being alone with my thoughts would not be wise. The weed wasn't numbing the pain any more – after smoking so much of it, I was growing immune. I needed a pick-me-up, desperately, so Natalie and I began to do a few lines of coke occasionally, with some dodgy 'friends' who sold the stuff. Coke did not help the physical pain in the slightest – if anything, it sharpened it – but it did make me feel slightly happier – enough to be able to enjoy myself when I was out. This is how it becomes addictive; it stops you feeling down, so you take more and more and then, before you know it, you're taking it all the time to cover up the emotional pain that you don't realise won't go away anyway. We loved it, it was a huge part of our lives and our evenings revolved around our next line or how we would get hold of another gram. Weed often made me feel deflated but coke, well, I just loved the feeling it gave me. We came up with code names for it, and because we liked drinking Archers and lemonade, we would refer to a gram of coke as a bottle of archers, or half a gram as half a bottle of archers. She'd text me saying, 'Got half a bottle of Archers for tonight.' I'd usually go round to her house first, do a few lines, then head on to meet the girls who had no idea we were doing it. Once, me and Natalie were sat in the back of Zoe's car while Zoe was driving on the way to our favourite club, CC, by Leicester Square, and Natalie got the small pack out of her pocket, took a heap of coke under her extremely long acrylic nail on her baby finger (which was how we always took our lines so that we didn't leave any evidence on tables or toilet seats), held it up to my nose and I snorted it up, then did the same to her nose, then we rubbed a bit on our gums. The music was so loud and Zoe was talking to Mia in the front and Nicole wasn't paying attention in the back and no one even noticed.

CC became our new hangout. We made many friends in the London club scene and our status went from 'Smirnoff ice and PVC skirts at Destiny', to 'cocaine and expensive clothes at CC'.

We knew the doormen, the bouncers, and the manager and walked straight past the long queue each time and straight into the club where we'd be escorted up to the VIP section and the table that was always reserved just for us. This was mainly because of some of our male friends who had connections and after a while, we were as known to the club as them.

Not one Saturday night went past without us going to CC. In the summer, we'd spend the day at Zoe's house by her pool, have a barbeque and get ready there, then go up to CC, then go back and sleep there if her parents were away, which was quite often. Otherwise, sometimes I'd go back and sleep at Natalie's and the sound of our incessant sniffing was enough to keep the whole house awake.

On New Years Eve 2001 or 2002 – I honestly couldn't tell you which one, they all morphed into one, big, coke-fuelled oblivion – Natalie and I went to pick up a few grams in the afternoon in preparation for our night out and on the way back, we got into a car accident. Natalie had only recently started driving and tended to be quite nervous. It didn't help that she hadn't spent much time at the wheel sober. But this accident wasn't her fault. We were driving along the main road that led to where we both lived and we saw a car that was parked, and looked like it was edging out. Natalie slowed down as we could see him moving but expected he'd wait until we passed as there wasn't enough time to let him out but he sped out anyway and went right into my side. We stopped and got out, I had really hurt my arm as the car basically went right into it and my head hit the dashboard. Natalie had also sprung forward quite forcefully but we seemed to be OK. The guy who hit us got out of his car and started shouting and screaming, then a bystander came along and said she witnessed it and saw that it was his fault. We were just outside Danielle's house and after hearing the commotion, Danielle's mum came outside. After the police had arrived and we had given our statement, and called our friend Craig to come down and meet us as we were going out with him that night and he lived a minute away, we went into Danielle's house and her mum gave us a cup of hot sweet tea. We left not long after and told everyone we were fine. We weren't fine, but we'd be damned if we missed out on snorting time on New Year's Eve. By half way through the night, we could barely move and we spent the whole of New Year's Day in Accident & Emergency, worried the whole time that blood tests would show the copious amounts of cocaine in our systems. It didn't, we got away with it, but we were in a state.

In the end, I received £2000 from insurance for that accident and kept it in a savings account and later bought my first car with it. Good car accident, in the end.

We spent a lot of time at Nick and Nick's, in Watford. They were friends of friends and they sold drugs, a lot. They lived in this dive of a house with about six other people and it was revolting but it was the only place Natalie and I could openly get high. Most times we'd go there after a night out but sometimes we'd just go round there in the middle of the day or early evening. One night after clubbing, we all went back there and just kept on doing line after line after line. We would cut lines that were really long on the mirrored tray and see who could snort the longest line without stopping. We did so much coke, followed by so much weed that night and I remember I kept saying, "I don't know what I am." What I meant by that was, I didn't know if I was buzzing from the coke or chilled from the weed. I was both. My body could barely move from being so stoned, by my mind was crazy and the seven of us (sometimes more), would sit around in the lounge having the world's deepest conversations about life and death and the world beyond and the meaning of life and other such subjects. Coke makes you want to talk and talk and get all your feelings out so when I was talking, if someone stopped me and gave their opinion or started saying something, I would cry, because I was so upset that I didn't get to finish off saying what I wanted to say.

Some days we'd go round there during the day and help The Nicks cut and pack their drugs. We'd sit there weighing each pack with garage music blaring in the background while we were all too stoned to even speak. Every so often The Nicks would go and get bags of food (and toilet paper, we always needed more toilet paper) and bring it back so we could eat but coke takes away your appetite so we barely ate at all. The Nicks were actually really nice. In a strange way we all really cared about each other. We would always be in touch during days we weren't together and the Nicks always made sure me and Natalie were OK, drinking enough water and were looked after. Funny really.

Just over a year after Natalie and I had started doing coke

together, she went away for a week with her mum and while she was away, I was asking some of the boys to get me some coke. When she came back she said that the boys had told her I was doing coke on my own, and that was something to be worried about (this coming from drug dealing addicts. Honourable I suppose, in a way). I was defensive at first, then I realised she was right. I was doing coke on my own? Was I a coke addict? No, I wasn't an addict, surely? I could give it up whenever I wanted, I just chose to carry on because it made me feel better. But even the Nicks were worried, which meant I came across as an addict and I knew in my heart that was not what I wanted for my life. Whatever I had been through or was still going through, I still believed that I was better than that, that I could be better than that, that life, somehow – and I wasn't sure how – would get better and there would be light at the end of that perennially dark tunnel.

I went home that day, got in the bath with a joint (which my parents ended up letting me do as I told them it helped the pain) and assessed my situation. I thought about it hard and deep and made a decision. I went round to Natalie's the next day and we both decided to stop doing coke.

I was eighteen. What decisions and choices I'd already had to make by the age of eighteen. And how many people can say that they had an addiction and beat it by the age of eighteen? It's crazy to look back while writing this book and assess all the things I've been through and all the things I've overcome; choices I made – both bad and good – without any guidance because I chose to separate myself from my parents. And although the initial choices I made led to the abhorrent situations I found myself in, I do believe my strong upbringing ultimately led me to the good decisions I eventually made. That, and a power from above trying, despite my desperate attempts to ignore the signs, to lead me in the right direction.

Natalie gave in on a couple of occasions and had a line here and there at parties but I never touched the stuff again. Most people start doing drugs at the age that I stopped and at eighteen I had given it up for good.

We agreed that this was just a secret part of our life, something that had helped us get through a difficult time and we did it together. We could put it down to experience. No one need ever know. But my nose was never the same...

My parents barely knew me anymore. I had turned into a monster that they couldn't control and with whom they had no relationship and I hated this. Despite my efforts to alienate myself from my 'actual' life, I never wanted to lose my parents – I loved the relationship I had with them, especially Mum. I was hiding so much from them and couldn't bring myself to get closer to them, in case I blurted it all out one day. I didn't want to be questioned, so I distanced myself.

Around this time, Nanny was diagnosed with breast cancer. I am sure that all the stress took its toll on Mum. Nanny had a lump removed and then weekly radiotherapy. Thank goodness, she recovered, but she was never really the same after that. I don't know how Mum dealt with it all. At the time I didn't think about how all of this affected her although, no matter what I was like with other things in my life, I was always there for Nanny and helped in any way I could, hoping they could see this.

My friends knew how depressed I was and I would speak about Michael occasionally but, as I couldn't really talk to anyone about my innermost thoughts, I started to write them down. I wrote diary entries and poems about how I was feeling and, while researching for this book, I found my diary and read what I had written over this two-year period. I hadn't realised it at the time, but I was seriously delusional. I had blocked out what Michael had done to me to such an extent that I believed I was in love with him. I obsessed over him and the baby that I had miscarried and, in between poems and diary entries about Michael, there was the occasional one about being in pain.

I had written a letter to Michael that I hadn't intended to give him, instead hoping that by writing down how I was feeling it would help. I put the letter in my diary.

One day, Mum called me when I was at my after-college telesales job, to say that she, not Aba, would pick me up. She sounded as if she was crying and I didn't understand why. The letter, which mentioned the miscarriage, had fallen out of my diary and Aba had picked it up and read it. When Mum picked me up from work, she looked at me with sadness washing over her face.

This huge thing had happened to me and they had known nothing about it; in fact, they thought I was still a virgin. Aba had been sick after reading the letter. I didn't want the homeward journey to end that day, as I didn't want to face him. It was that unexplainable feeling where you just wish more than anything that you could turn back time and change things, that if you could, you could fix things. I couldn't believe that I had managed to cause my parents so much distress when I never meant to be so rebellious. Aba couldn't even look at me. I had no choice but to explain the situation to Mum. She said that she didn't know what to feel any more, that she was void of all feeling and that I wasn't the same person she once knew. And I wasn't. Even then, when I had the opportunity to open up, I couldn't tell her what had happened the night that led to me being pregnant. I told her the same story that I had told the doctor. Mum left me in my room that night crying my eyes out, and I heard her doing the same from across the hall.

A few weeks later, my cousin Shimon in South Africa offered to send a ticket for me to come and stay with him for a couple of weeks. We agreed that this had come at just the right time. My family was going to Israel for Passover and I would be in South Africa, and I desperately hoped that this would make me feel better. None of us really knew how to deal with what was going on with me. Mum and Aba could barely even look at me, so going abroad for a fresh break seemed like a wise option. I hoped that it would make me feel happier and also hoped that somehow, when I returned, I could rebuild my relationship with Mum again. I missed her.

I had been smoking so much weed for so long that the flight to South Africa nearly killed me. It was bad enough that I had insomnia at home but an eleven-hour flight without any weed or cigarettes was unbearable. I had lost all sense of time and didn't know when or if we would ever land. Eventually, of course, we did land and I spent the time in South Africa relaxing and trying to move on from the whirlwind of the past year. As I couldn't get hold of any weed out there, I made a conscious effort to stop altogether. For the first few days I sweated a lot and was jumpy and couldn't sleep, but being in the heat and in a different environment and around nature soon changed things and I felt refreshed and renewed. When I came back, I never smoked it again.

I didn't change straight away. Michael eventually got back in touch and over the following year I saw him on and off. Don't ask me why – I don't know the answer. I was possessed, still not really the Lauren I wanted to be or knew I was. The group dynamic had changed by this time; Marina had moved back to Bulgaria and the girls were getting tired of my anger problems, not knowing how to cope with them anymore. We began to argue and, every so often, Lana would call a 'meeting', where the six of us would meet at the Elstree Moat House bar to talk things through.

Eventually, I came to realise that it was not just my family that was bearing the brunt of my anger, it was my friends too, so I was sent to anger management sessions. Funnily enough, the only thing that stopped me being so angry and made me see the light regarding Michael was the one thing that I had spent all this time running away from…

Chapter 6

Till the End of Time

Anger management didn't change anything profoundly, but it did help me to understand myself more, and more significantly, to understand where the anger was coming from and why. Writing it down now makes it seem so simple to work out but, at the time, I had no idea why I was so angry, I'm not even sure I knew that I *was* angry.

The sweet, petite, mocha-skinned therapist worked out that one of the main things that I was frustrated about, was other people not understanding the extent of my pain. This is why I took so much anger out on my friends. Although I now had a very close group of friends who were always there for me, they never really understood. But then again, I didn't really talk about it either, I'd just been doing drugs to cover it up and doing anything and everything possible to not face the arthritis. Anger management taught me something simple yet effective: they don't understand because they've never been through it themselves, so how can they understand? My friends will never know what it feels like to have arthritis, but they were trying, and I had to accept this and move on. And if I wanted them to understand as much as was possible for them, I had to talk about it sometimes.

Realising what it was that was making me angry all this

time became the first step towards bringing me back to my old self. The realisation itself had an enormous impact on the way I thought about things. It may sound ridiculous now, when my story is written in black and white, from beginning to end, and so what was making me feel like that is quite obvious, but at the time, I couldn't see beyond what was going on in my head and couldn't bring myself to face the past, and although I did face the past to some extent, my first step towards healing came from focusing on the present and how to move forward, not spend my time focusing on what had already happened.

I had to admit how I felt. So how did I feel? I was angry with God for giving me arthritis, I was angry at the fact that my childhood revolved around it, I was trying to deal with losing the sight in my eye, I couldn't walk very well and I felt that my future was taken out of my hands and I had no way of having any say over what my future would hold. So no biggie then, just a few minor issues for an eighteen year old to trawl through.

Somehow, despite my two years of irrational, and quite frankly revolting, behaviour, I passed my college exams with Distinction and there were many options open to me, or there would have been were I able to make long-term commitments. In the midst of my drug addiction, anger issues and burgeoning disability, along with the rest of the absurdity of the past few years that at the time was one big blur, I had still applied to study acting and directing at a few universities. I completed the arduous task of filling in the dreaded UCAS forms and went along to auditions and interviews. During one of my visits to a university (I can't remember which one it was), Natalie came with and while walking around and assessing the students and their accommodation, we decided that if I did end up going there, she'd come with me and we'd sell weed (this was before we gave up coke). Seemed like a no-brainer. All the students smoked and we could get hold of it. Just another one of our brilliant ideas.

Anyway, I got offered a few places, including LIPA (The Liverpool Institute for Performing Arts) which is one of the best in the country, Bath University and, shockingly, the highly respected Italia Conti Academy of Theatre Arts. Italia Conti was only offering me a one year foundation course but not on a scholarship, I'd have to pay for it in full. (My audition piece for Italia Conti was my favourite Lady Jane Grey monologue, of course.) If I had a clearer head I probably would have recognised that this was one of the best things that could have happened to me, it was God's way of saying 'here we go, I'm giving you a break, take it'. Getting into Italia Conti, even if I wasn't offered a scholarship or a three year degree, was a real achievement and could have put me in touch with the right people and got my foot in the door for the following years, but all I could think at the time was, 'well I can't afford to pay for it, can't ask my parents to get a loan for it, and what's the point of doing a one year course to then have to start a three year course afterwards. May as well save myself the time and go straight to the degree course elsewhere. That's if I can even walk by then.' This pretty much summed up my attitude at the time: defeatist. But as I started off this chapter talking about how not to regret the past and how to simply face the future, I will try my hardest now not to be bitter about that choice – the only regret I think I really have in life – as I write this, ten years later... Sorry, you'll have to give me a moment while I try hard not to be bitter...

Taking Italia Conti out the picture, which is what I seemed to do quite effortlessly (I didn't even reply to their letter), I was left with the options of LIPA and Bath. Both offered everything I was looking for, apart from the fact that they were both ridiculously far away from London, and I could get a student loan for either which I couldn't do with Italia Conti as it was foundation. Both courses meant I could study the directing side whilst learning about drama and still get to act. Everyone I knew was going to Leeds, Manchester or Birmingham and, although part of me wanted to be around people I knew, I thought that getting away from everyone I knew would be what I needed most. I knew that in order to perfect my craft I needed to know everything and have a back-up plan if acting didn't work. I'd always been interested in directing and I was really looking forward to studying the intricacies of film making. I also knew that throwing myself totally into something I loved, without any other distractions, would help me put the past behind me.

My health, however, was all over the place. The timing was off. How could I locate myself four hours from home when I was in so much pain and it was just getting worse? Mum said that I had too many hospital appointments and we needed to figure something out first so, after much contemplation, I decided to defer entry for both LIPA and Bath for a year in order to get my health back in order. This way, I thought that by the time I did go to university the following year, my head would be in a much better place. I had been looking forward to everything uni had to offer but I knew I'd enjoy it more if I was healthy and in a better place emotionally. Being away from home wouldn't have been easy. I also thought that it gave me an opportunity to get a job for a year and earn some money to help me out with my student loan as my parents weren't in a position to help me out.

I got a job as a junior lettings agent in an estate agency in Edgware called Kramer Estates.

I was quite good at the job. Selling came naturally to me, even though I didn't particularly enjoy it. After a few months I was head-hunted by an agency round the corner called Melvin Jacobs. Simon, my boss, told me that if I worked hard enough, I could do very well in property and even have my own property by the time I was twenty-one. Although this sounded like a great prospect, and it was actually quite appealing to see myself as a high-flying professional with my own property, I just didn't see myself working in an office for the rest of my life and my plan was still to go to uni but everything was changing.

Something shifted in the dynamic between Michael and me. He was more needy, trying, so he said, to change his life and get a proper job blah blah blah, and he relied on me to help him. But it was extreme, he literally couldn't move an inch without calling me and getting my approval. He needed me for everything and I liked that at the beginning, it was like I had won, like after all this time of fighting, the tables had turned and he needed me like I had needed him. But I didn't want to be the girl who stuck by this idiot while he tried to change his life because despite everything, I was clever enough to know that he would never really change his life or be the kind of person I knew I wanted for myself, he didn't have the capacity for change, or the intelligence to do anything more with his life and I knew that the person he was, went deeper than a job or a house, he'd always just be the asshole who pushed over an old man at Edgware station. He started turning up at my work and calling my work phone all the time and my colleagues thought he was harassing me. It got to the point where I couldn't even bear to look at him; I didn't want to be around him anymore. I just wanted so desperately to be my old self again, and this is what gave me the strength. I'd said in one of the poems I'd written that the one thing I'd never be able to do would be to walk away knowing the hold he'd always had over me, but I knew I had to, and I now felt like I had the strength. We met one evening and whilst sitting in the passenger seat of his Jeep I told him that it was over for good and not to contact me ever again. He seemed genuinely upset, or as genuine as someone like him could be, and tried to contact me a few times, but I changed my phone number and felt as if a weight had been lifted from my shoulders. At the time, I felt that cutting him off was the hardest thing I'd ever done, but I finally knew, deep down, that it was for the best. Best for my emotional health, my physical health, my family and for my friendships.

In time, I slowly began to rebuild the relationship with my parents, who I think were trying to regain their trust in me but were walking on eggshells around me in case 'the monster' in me should reappear. At the same time, they were extremely worried about my deteriorating health.

Mum suggested that we go back to the Homeopathic Centre in Edgware to see if Vicky was still there. I had started seeing Vicky, who was a homeopath, after Beatrice left the clinic and I saw her monthly for a few years until I was about twelve. We walked in and Ian, the lovely man whom we'd met all those years before, was still there standing behind the counter. He explained that Vicky had moved to Kent, but there was a new homeopath there, called Lubina.

Although Mum came with me to the first session with Lubina, I went in to see her on my own, as I was older now and she needed to really get to know me. I don't know what it was about Lubina, but I felt a very strong connection with her. I was able to open up to her more than I did with anyone else. She was not only my homeopath, but my counsellor. Just talking to her made me feel better and I started believing she was sent to me for a reason.

Lubina was originally from India and still had a slight accent. She had a beautiful face and warm, dark eyes that made me feel welcome. She always wore nice clothes and open shoes or sandals, which showed off her immaculately pedicured feet. I would chat with her for about forty minutes and then lie on the bed, where she would give me Life Force Healing, which I suppose could be compared today to Craniosacral Therapy. It was very much like the spiritual healing I had had when I was younger. Life force healing restores the natural flow of energy, allowing the body to heal itself. I believed in homeopathy and healing and the meaning behind them and I always trusted them more than conventional medicine but had yet to find my way with it all and understand it properly.

Lubina spent a lot of time working on my eye and kept saying that not only was I very blocked, but there were things I didn't want to 'see' and this needed to be worked out before the eye could get better. By not telling anyone about what Michael had done, I had not accepted or dealt with it in the slightest. I didn't believe that it had happened, so this didn't even occur to me when Lubina asked what it was that I didn't want to 'see'. I only wish I had worked it out then. There were other factors too, which only came to light many years later.

At the last hospital appointment with Dr. Graham, she had said that if my health continued to deteriorate, I would have to consider medication. We'd always been very much against conventional medications and I'd been lucky to stay away from them so far, but now things were becoming tricky. I went to my next appointment at St Thomas' with Mum and we spoke to Dr. Graham about the options. We had discussed a particular drug, which I will call M, before. I was offered this drug when I was seven but at the time it was still an experimental drug and the doctors wanted to use me to trial it. Obviously, my parents had been against this and so I never took it. But now it was now fully 'approved' and was given to children with cancer and people with auto-immune diseases like arthritis.

M is a very strong drug and works by inhibiting the activity in the immune system to cut down the amount of inflammation that is produced. Dr. Graham explained this to us but, at the time, I couldn't take it all in and Mum asked most of the questions. The doctor discussed the side effects, but explained that serious ones, such as liver and kidney damage, were rare and not everyone experienced the other side effects. Nausea was the first one that she mentioned. If she had wanted to put me off, using the word 'nausea' was the right way to go about it with someone who had a phobia of vomiting. It was bad enough that I had to take a drug like this, the last thing I wanted was to be sick the whole time that I was on it.

Dr. Graham had convinced me that my eye was getting so inflamed that soon I would have no vision at all, and then there would be nothing more they could do. We needed to take drastic action; there were no more options and not enough time. Dr. Smith had also advised that M would radically help the arthritis. She told me that most of the people I knew from physiotherapy were all taking it and although there could be some side effects, it worked for 70% of patients. What I didn't ask at the time was, what did they mean by 'worked'? Because their version of a drug working and my version of a drug working were two exponentially different things.

Mum was against it from the outset, but I needed something to stop the pain and help my eye. I thought that if I took the medication just until the inflammation had gone down in the eye, this would give us enough time to operate on the cataract and then I could come off the drug. Mum wasn't convinced, but she decided that as I was now an adult, I had to make this decision for myself, and so I did. We arranged to go back to St Thomas' to receive my first dose of treatment. There was an option to take it in a weekly injection but I would be taking it in tablet form once a week with folic acid. Once a week didn't sound too bad.

Luckily, it was now 2002 and the Internet helped us to research the medication but I'm not sure this was such a good thing at the time. If we weren't scared before we certainly were now. The side effects sounded dreadful; worse than the doctors had made out. It appeared that it could cause severe toxicity of the liver, kidneys and bone marrow and this should be monitored by monthly blood tests. More common side effects included ulcers (anywhere, not just in the mouth), stomach upset and nausea, low white blood counts, headaches, dizziness, fatigue, itchiness and rashes and, worst of all, hair loss.

Lubina had her reservations, of course, but she said that if I'd made up my mind to take the drug we could carry on with the homeopathy alongside it and she would give me something to prevent the sickness. It probably seems quite trivial to you that I was worried about feeling sick when there were so many other side-effects to worry about but I just couldn't bear the thought of being sick.

I spoke to my friends about what would be happening and told them I'd probably be slowed down a bit and wouldn't be able to go clubbing as much and I wouldn't be able to drink alcohol. They were all supportive but I'm not sure they quite understood the significance of an eighteen year old starting a chemo-based drug.

Nicole, who had lost the 'Ni' from the beginning of her name and was now affectionately known as 'Cole', ever the mother hen of the group, decided to go off and do her own research into M. Although I had discovered the same things as her, I took comfort in knowing that she cared enough to take the time out to understand what I'd be going through. She was the only one out of all of them who ever really got the significance of it and who made allowances for my physical shortcomings. Once I started getting ill, they all stopped inviting me out because they just assumed I wouldn't want to go. Cole was the only one who'd still call and tell me what the plans were to try and include me.

Natalie, Zoe and I decided to go all out and book a really

crazy holiday to Cancun in Mexico and I told Dr. Graham I'd start taking M when I got back. I needed one last bit of freedom to enjoy first.

Zoe was now going out with Craig and he and all his friends had booked to come too, although they were staying in a different hotel. I had a job so I was able to afford to save up for it (and it's amazing how much money you're able to save when you're not spending it on coke). We spent fifteen days in an all-inclusive resort and I still believe it to have been the best holiday of my life. I felt ready to get back and start M. But our holiday was to be tainted with the most awful news when we returned.

Our flight back to London had been delayed by a few hours and our baggage did not arrive with our flight, so when we got off the plane we had to wait in the baggage reclaim area for hours. While we were waiting, I received a phone call from Mum. She asked if Natalie could overhear what she was saying. Very gently, Mum said, "Please don't act as though you are shocked and don't act like I have told you anything, for Natalie's sake, but there has been an accident." I didn't know what to think: was it her parents? Her sister? "Jake has been in car accident. He's… dead." My heart sank. She couldn't have been serious. Jake? Couldn't be. He's only twenty-one, I thought. I wanted to ask questions, and then I wanted to cry but somehow, I kept calm.

Natalie's parents wanted to tell her the news. They had arranged to have her mobile phone cut off, so that messages about Jake wouldn't get through to her while she was on holiday. We heard on the 15th July and he had died three days earlier. I needed to tell somebody, so I managed to get Zoe to accompany me to the toilet so that I could share the news. I needed to – I was shaking and shuddering and didn't know how to feel, but I did know that Natalie would be utterly devastated and we had to keep it from her until she arrived home.

Zoe and I had agreed that we'd go home, dump our cases and wait for the call from Natalie's mum to tell us it was OK to go over. I knew I had to put my feelings to one side, because although Jake had meant a lot to me, Natalie had been with him for three years. She was going to be devastated. She never really accepted or acknowledged that that I'd had a relationship with him. Out of all the myriad things that Natalie and I spoke about, especially during nights when we were high on coke and up until the morning spilling our hearts out to each other, it was one thing we never spoke about. I cried in my bedroom, not really knowing how to feel, then washed my face and put on a brand new one for Natalie. Zoe and I arrived at her house, only an hour later and after travelling for fifteen hours, and she didn't seem too bad. She didn't know what to say or how to accept it, but I guess none of us did.

After Natalie and Jake had broken up, they hadn't had any contact and he had eventually moved back to Derby, where his family lived. The hardest thing to accept was that we never had the chance to say goodbye. The three of us, with Natalie's mum and stepdad – who had hated Jake, but kept quiet now – sat in their kitchen drinking tea and smoking cigarettes for the rest of the day. We tried to talk about it but all that really came out of our ramblings was that we couldn't believe or accept that he was gone.

Jake's funeral took place two weeks later in Derby. Tarek had arranged a coach to take everyone up there but, aside from the fact that I knew Michael was going to be on the coach and I didn't want to be anywhere near him, my legs were now too stiff to sit on a coach for long, so Cole offered to drive me along with Zoe and another friend.

Cole, aside from being a mother hen is also a 'rules' girl, and followed her mother's instructions to not drive any faster than sixty miles per hour and to stay in the middle lane, and then we got lost, so we missed the service at the Church and I was utterly devastated. We made it to the burial ground, but when I heard that during the service they had played Tupac's Till the End of Time', I was even more upset as Tupac was *our* thing, *our* connection. The burial ground was on a beautiful hill and was very peaceful, but everyone was crying. I still felt that I had to hold it together for Natalie, so I stood alone weeping to myself. Some of the girls saw, and after everyone had left for the Wake, they helped me back up the hill and stood with me while I cried out loud.

I had never been to a Wake before. It was a strange experience. I wasn't used to watching people getting drunk and having a party after someone had died, but Jake's life deserved to be celebrated and, if this is what they were doing, then I was happy.

At the Wake, something occurred to me. I asked Tarek if he remembered the conversation in his car the first day I had met Jake, when Jake had said how strongly he felt a connection to Tupac, knowing that he would die early, just like him. He had said that he would be lucky if he made it to his twenty-first birthday.

Well, he did make it to his twenty-first birthday and died four months later. He was clearly more intuitive than any of us had given him credit for. How under-estimated his abilities had been. Jake could have been something in this life but had been dealt a bad hand. Despite everything he got up to, he had a good heart and deserved to be remembered in that way.

The next few weeks were strange. It hurt to think that Jake was gone and that I would never say goodbye. He may have been a rogue, but he was there for me when I was having the hardest time. He was the one who insisted on taking me straight to the doctor when I was having the miscarriage, the only one who genuinely cared what happened to me, apart from Cole, of course. Jake was more intelligent than he made out and he understood people's emotions better than most. I think, deep down, that he knew my pain and, although we were together, he knew my pain was because of Michael and in those short few months he never left me alone with my thoughts. He knew what damage Michael had done to me emotionally and how self-conscious I had become because of it, and he tried to make me feel better about myself at any opportunity.

After Jake's passing, nothing was ever the same. The group had split. We didn't see the boys any more – it was too hard. I still saw Tarek, but only on my own, because having a whole group of people there too would have made Jake's absence more painful. I spent a lot of time with Kate, whose boyfriend, Ruben, had been one of Jake's best friends. Kate was always there when I needed to talk and always acknowledged my connection to Jake. Ruben always spoke about Jake in a positive way, which I loved. Natalie never spoke about Jake again.

Chapter 7

Fighting the Enemy

My life was a total mess. As hard as it was to deal with Jake's untimely death, as well as everything else that had happened in the past two years, I had to focus on getting better. My life wasn't going to wait for me, I was just going to keep getting older and life would pass me by if I didn't sort myself out. Plus I wanted the old me back and needed to prove to Mum that she was still there... somewhere.

I made a conscious effort to leave past events in the past and focus on this new chapter in my life. I went with Mum back to St Thomas' to see Dr. Graham, where she went over everything again and gave me one month's supply of M and folic acid. I was to come back once a month for check-ups and blood tests, and would have to take the medication for a minimum of three months to see any results. The doctors wanted me to take it for a year. I figured I could take it for a few months, get the inflammation down enough to be able to remove the cataract, and then come off the medication. I felt confident that this plan would work and, by the time the year was over, I would be cataract-free, walking without crutches and on my way to uni. Suffice to say, that was the last time I ever made a 'plan' for my health.

As my health deteriorated and the decision was made to

take M, I told my boss that I may be slowed down a bit but assured him that I would do my best to avoid it affecting my work. I was already finding it difficult to do a number of things that most people saw as normal: sitting at a desk, for instance. My legs became uncomfortable and sore – especially in the winter – and I felt so cold that I would spend most of the day sitting on top of the radiator taking my calls.

I began taking the pills the day after my appointment at St. Thomas'. With homeopathy, sometimes health gets worse before it gets better, because the homeopathy brings the illness out of the system and the patient feels the illness before it goes away. I thought that this must be happening with M, because very rapidly I started to feel ill. It felt as if I could feel the effects as soon as the tablet went down my throat.

I started off on a very small dose of 2.5mg, just one tablet, but it is amazing just how strong one small pill can be. I could taste the chemicals and feel them seeping into my bloodstream. I hated the fact I was taking it but just wanted it to work quickly so my life could go back to normal.

Because my grandparents were spiritualists, Mum had always had a strong belief in healing and had taken me to see a healer when I was younger.

Ray was a psychic surgeon who went into trance when healing, allowing the spirit of a doctor named Paul to enter his body, giving him the ability to heal people with his hands. For the skeptics and cynics among you, I appreciate how far-fetched this sounds. But I loved going to my healing sessions, they were so peaceful, and even if it doesn't work, the placebo effect never hurt anyone. And just to clarify, I do personally believe in it.

Ray worked mostly from the home of a lovely, beautifully spoken, gentle lady called Carol. She lived five minutes away in Mill Hill, in a huge and beautifully decorated house. She loved fairies and dragons and the whole house was adorned with pictures, paintings and ornaments. Carol had two Siamese cats that I found scary, probably because they reminded me of the evil Siamese cats from Lady and the Tramp.

The healing was done in a very peaceful room downstairs. I wished that the homeopath's room had been as welcoming. There were pictures of fairies everywhere and Carol would tell me their names. I believed that they were helping Ray to heal me. Mum always said that she could feel the power of the healing in that room. Once, she saw actual steam – which we believe to be the energy – coming out of the head of another healer, Alan, who was there helping Ray. Believing in something beyond what we could see or feel always helped me and I think it helped Mum too to know that there was another 'force' helping.

Mum's best friend, Jojo, is also a healer and she started healing at The Sanctuary in Southgate. By the time I starting taking M, we hadn't been back to Carol's since I was about eight so Jojo suggested that we give healing a try again and so we began to go there on Sunday afternoons.

It was the most bizarre experience to be there, but relaxing and somehow invigorating at the same time. It was a large house used solely for healing. While you wait to see the healer, you sit in the sitting room, a large room with comfortable chairs that looks out onto a beautiful garden. The secretary advises you to close your eyes and relax or meditate, taking off your shoes to relax you further and make you more grounded.

Nanny used to come with us and we would sit in that room together. After the healing session, I would go into a small, dark and very warm room, where I had to wait for at least five minutes, if not more, to allow the healing to take effect. Every time I went in and sat on the rocking chair, I would cry uncontrollably. Perhaps the healing released some deep emotions, or maybe I just felt that it was fine to cry in there but, for whatever reason, it happened every time.

By the time I reached the end of the three-month minimum time period for the drug I was on, I was really ill. The doctors had continued to increase the dosage and I had gone from taking 2.5mg to 30mg. I could barely eat, as everything made me feel sick, and whatever I did eat made my stomach bloat to the point that I looked pregnant. I was constantly tired and irritable and I could have slept at any point in the day (a great change from the insomnia that had plagued me the year before). I had at least two mouth ulcers at any time, although apparently I was lucky, as one of the other girls had them in unimaginable places. I often felt dizzy and disorientated and, when this happened, I had to shut my eyes and go to sleep. Most shockingly, I woke up some mornings to find clumps of my hair all over my pillow. I would rub my hands through my hair to check what was happening, but this only made more hair fall out. I didn't have cancer, so why did I have go through all this? Why was I taking a chemo-based drug when only a few years before I was pain free? I never lost all of my hair – thank goodness – probably about half of it I reckon. I know it isn't the end of the world, but on top of feeling so ill, it was not helping my morale.

Working eventually – and inevitably – became impossible as my joints got worse and worse and my energy levels dropped dramatically. I tried to keep going for as long as I could, but eventually I just couldn't do it anymore. I could no longer get out of bed in the morning let alone spend eight hours a day in an office and out at viewings. After eight months of working in property and only a few months after starting M, I had to give up my job.

About a month afterwards, Zoe, Nicole and a few of the boys decided to take a random trip to Brighton one weekend and asked me if I wanted to come. I was feeling so ill that I had stopped going out and spent most of my time at home. I didn't give them an answer until the very last minute, but Mum encouraged me to go, pointing out that having something else to focus on might make me feel better. I'd become a recluse because I couldn't bear the thought of being around anyone who couldn't understand the severity of my pain. They would get on with their normal lives and no one would be there to worry about me in the same way my mum did, and I couldn't handle that as I just needed home comforts. In the end I did go, but once we arrived and the girls were getting ready to go out, all I wanted to do was sleep. They tried to wake me up so we could go to a club, but I couldn't muster up the energy to go. It was so frustrating because, like any eighteen year-old, I wanted to go out and do all the fun things my friends were doing. Mostly I didn't want to miss out but I was too ill. I could hear everything that was going on around me, the girls rushing around the room getting ready, playing music and talking about boys, but I literally could not move. I felt as if I was on another planet.

I don't think the girls realised just how bad I was feeling, because when I said I couldn't get up and go to the club, Zoe got angry with me. She didn't understand that when I said I didn't have the energy to go out, I literally did not have any energy. This drug was not a joke; it was a seriously strong drug and it made me even more angry at my friends for not getting the severity of what was going on. The fact that Zoe was able to get angry at me just made me burn with rage. It was the exact reason I didn't want to go in the first place.

Later on that evening, while the girls were out and I was asleep in the hotel room, one of the boys we had come with, Jay, called me to say that he and his friends had decided to drive home that night and offered me a lift. I got into the back of Jay's car and went to sleep. Zoe was angry with me for several days and I couldn't understand why. Could she not see how ill I was? It was beyond me.

This was the only time that Zoe and I ever argued and we sorted it out within a few days, but it did make me realise where my frustrations about people not understanding came from. No matter how ill I've been, I have never wished that feeling on anyone, but sometimes I wanted my friends to feel as I did for just one day so that they would understand. I can see that this was probably quite selfish of me. It wasn't as if I wanted sympathy, quite the opposite. In fact, I would tell them to stop asking how I was on a daily basis to save me talking about it and would ask them to tell me about their problems instead. All I wanted was understanding.

By this point, the pain in my joints was unbearable. I could barely bend my knees because of the swelling and my ankles were so stiff that I couldn't put my feet in the position to walk properly. Knee and ankle pain were things I had experienced before. Pain in the rest of my body, however, was not something I was used to.

During the days when I was at home on my own, I had nothing to keep me occupied except my music and I remembered how much joy the guitar had given me when I was younger. I had nothing to do, I thought, so why not give it another go? I had all the time in the world to re-teach myself and maybe it would be a distraction from the pain. So I bought a 'teach yourself guitar' book and picked up my beautiful guitar as if I had never put it down. There was one problem. I hadn't realised that I had arthritis in my hands.

Out of nowhere, I was experiencing the arthritis pain in my hands that had been so familiar in my knees and ankles and, within a matter of a few short months, it had spread to my hips, feet, elbows, shoulders, wrists, neck and jaw. I was now arthritic from head to toe.

Just like that, I couldn't sit properly, because bending my

hips was too painful. I couldn't hold the phone to my ear, or brush my teeth, because my elbows wouldn't bend and my fingers were too swollen to grip. I couldn't chew food because my jaw was stiff and I couldn't walk because my knees, ankles and feet were in constant pain. It was hard to take in the fact that, after all the years of having arthritis in my knees and ankles and one small tendon in my left hand, all of a sudden, within the space of a few months, it was everywhere. Playing the guitar certainly wasn't an option now.

Daily tasks became impossible. I couldn't put on my own socks and shoes because that involved far too many joints and I couldn't tie my shoelaces. I completely lost my independence, even needing help in the bathroom. Mum took me to the toilet, pulled down my knickers and then pulled them back up for me. She had to help me in and out of the bath and brush my teeth and hair for me. She shaved my legs and under my arms and dried me after my bath. I lost all dignity.

The worst bit was not being able to feed myself. I felt like a baby, or a quadriplegic, needing someone to do everything for me, including spooning food into my mouth. Anything I drank had to come out of a straw, because I couldn't lift the glass or manoeuvre it enough to get the liquid in my mouth.

Despite my frustrations, Mum was amazing. Anything she could do, she did. When you cannot do anything yourself, you realise how much you actually do. Simple tasks like getting a drink, going to the toilet, turning on the TV or taking a shower all required someone else's help and I felt as if I was spending all day every day calling Mum into my room to help me. She worked most days, so we had to do the showering in the morning before she left. Aba was at home during the day to help with the other stuff.

When I was younger, I was given lessons by my physiotherapists on how to use crutches properly. For instance, if no one was around and I had to use the stairs, I wouldn't be able to use both crutches because I needed to hold onto the banister. They taught me how to hold onto the banister with my left hand and, with one crutch in my right hand, I would angle the other under the fingers of the same hand and hop up the stairs. This is perfect when it is just your legs that hurt, but there are no lessons that can show you what to do when you can't use both arms and both legs. So I perfected 'the bum shuffle'.

I went back to Middlesex Hospital in a wheelchair and Dr. Smith called out for "*Laura* Vaknine." Was she being serious?? I had been a patient of hers for years and she couldn't even do me the decency of remembering my name. Apart from that, she did not seem at all fazed by the fact that Mum was pushing me into her room in a wheelchair. She was a paediatric rheumatologist; where the hell was her bedside manner?!

Dr. Smith loved to talk about coincidences. This was no coincidence. For sixteen years I had had arthritis in just five joints and, after ten months of taking this drug, I had it everywhere. No, this was definitely not a coincidence; M had reacted to my body in an awful way and no one paid any attention to how bad it was getting. Not Dr. Smith, not the physiotherapists and not Dr. Graham. Why could no one see how rapidly my health was deteriorating?

All Dr. Smith could say was that M worked for 70% of patients and did not work for the other 30%, into which percentage I fell. "I am not a statistic. I am me," I shouted, my voice breaking. "I have a name and it is not *Laura* and if you can't do me the courtesy of remembering that after so many years and all you've put me through then I want to be referred to another rheumatologist." Did they not realise that everyone was different? That perhaps I fell into a totally different category and they should try and work out what it was that was causing this horrific reaction? No. No one tried to figure anything out, they just stuck me into their little category and left it at that.

I burst into tears and Mum tried to calm me down. She knew that I was right and felt as I did, but she asked me in a whisper not to be rude. I didn't care if I was being rude. I was so upset and frustrated and shouted at the doctor for allowing my life to become like this, for letting me end up in a wheelchair with arthritis from head to toe and half a head of hair, at only nineteen years old.

In my frenetic state I told Dr. Smith that, now my year's trial was nearly over (it had been ten months) and I was a hundred times worse than I was before, with no opportunity whatsoever to have my eye operated upon, I wanted to come off the drug. I had to be weaned off it slowly and knew that coming off a strong drug too quickly could be dangerous, but other than the information she was reeling off about the weaning, I barely listened to her ramblings.

All these strong drugs ever do is suppress the symptoms, but they don't seem to deal with the root problem. Mum had been right all this time to keep me on homeopathy, because this boosted my immune system and allowed my body to fight the illness. When taking strong drugs, the body is not strong enough to fight anything and so everything shuts down and, for me, the drug didn't even help the symptom it was supposed to be helping! Later, I would learn that I had to stop trying to fight my illness so hard, in order for it to go away. It started to make me think about drugs and illnesses and how they were treated. I began wondering how an illness can be treated if the root problem isn't tackled? This is what Mum had thought all along, but I was so used to everyone else making decisions for me from a young age that I never questioned these decisions – until I was offered M and thought why not, maybe it can help. I hadn't had the time to realise for myself that Mum had always been right. Perhaps I needed to have had my own experience of making the wrong decision to really understand what Mum had felt all these years.

It was not the drug itself that I was angry with, it was the fact that the doctors did not monitor what it was doing to me personally, that the system was set up in a way to benefit the pharmaceutical companies and not the patients. Yes, they took their monthly blood tests but what was going on in front of their eyes was not even considered. I felt that all these doctors were too quick to put vulnerable people on strong drugs, making them feel that there is no other way, then use labs and tests to do the work for them instead of looking into the eyes of the patient to see what was really going on, or was that too easy for people who had been to medical school? My frustration with the medical establishment was extreme, because I felt that they couldn't look past their statistics to see what was sitting in front of them. Everyone is different and everyone reacts differently to medications but they pay no attention to this because making millions of drugs for one illness won't benefit the pharmaceutical companies. Homeopathy believes in treating the person, not the disease and, for me, this made so much more sense. I suppose that, after many years of being treated with alternative therapies, my body may have thrown out the drug because it wasn't used to anything chemical, in the same way that if you gave a chemical that strong to an indigenous people who had never ingested anything but natural goodness, their bodies would do the same. But that wasn't all there was to it, what I am writing now was just my thinking at the time. I had yet to learn many lessons and I will get to them...

Mum got me a strawberry Ribena, my favourite drink – and perhaps the wrong thing to be having considering the sugar and artificial crap in it – on the way out of the clinic and tried to calm me down in the car, but all I could do was cry.

Mum reminded me about a girl we had met in hospital who had recommended another Rheumatologist. April was a couple of years older than me and had the same type of arthritis. She had taken the conventional route throughout her whole life, and had a puffy face from steroids and a few joint deformities. When I saw her, and the hundreds of others who walked through the hospital like her, it was the only time I felt lucky. Regardless of what I was going through, the fact that I'd never taken steroids and had only had ten months on M, meant that I looked normal and even if I was in pain, this is of utmost importance to a nineteen year old.

I had originally met April and her mother in the waiting room at St Thomas', as she also had uveitis and was in my hydro group at Northwick Park.

I began to enjoy hydro a bit more as I had now been assigned to a new physiotherapist, Andre. Andre made everything fun for me again, even though during our one-to-one physio sessions, he pushed my pain to the limit. He would try to get my joints moving again and I would sometimes hit him as a reflex when it really hurt, but he took it well and made me try harder. At that point, he was the one physio, in fact, the one person who worked in a hospital, who tried to know me as me. I felt comfortable with him, because he asked me about my life in a way that only my homeopaths had done up until then. This changed when I met Dr. Keat.

Dr. Andrew Keat was the Rheumatologist who April and her mother had told us about in the waiting room outside Dr. Graham's clinic. April had also been with Dr. Smith and was then transferred to Dr. Keat at Northwick Park. She said that he was fantastic and much more understanding than many of the other doctors she had come across. We sent a letter to my Rheumatologist asking her for a transfer and luckily we got one. It was also much more convenient for us to get to

Northwick Park.

I saw April at hydro once a week and, although it was nice to be friends with someone who understood my pain, I didn't want to be around other 'arthritis people'. At hydro sessions, all anyone spoke about was arthritis and it actually made me feel worse than I was. Granted, at this point, it couldn't really get much worse, but at least when I was with my own friends, I felt semi-normal and that I belonged somewhere other than in an arthritis network and that arthritis was something I had, not something I was.

When I was with other arthritics, we were in 'Arthritis World', and this made me feel as if it was my only world and I didn't want that. When something becomes such a big part of your life, it seems bigger than it is and I wasn't prepared to sink into that, I wasn't prepared to be known as 'Lauren from Arthritis group.' So, when April asked if I wanted to join her and some of the others on one of the 'arthritis days out', I instantly declined. That was all I needed – to sit on a bus that was full of disabled people, all comparing medications and ESRs, and then get off the bus at a farm or something equally as generic, while people stared at us sympathetically. No, I would rather stay home and watch The OC, thanks.

Mum tried many different methods to get me well again. Anything that she heard about that might work, she bought me. She bought me a copper bracelet as recommended by a man we'd met on holiday. I didn't really find that it helped, although I could see that the concept behind it made sense. After a month, Mum came across a stall in the Broadwalk that was selling 'special' magnetic copper bracelets for £120, and she bought one for me. All her spare money went on me. We placed our vitamins on a tray in the kitchen and Mum now filled this tray with natural remedies she had found. Over the years she accumulated cod liver oil, glucosamine, omega 3, Korean red ginseng, flax seed oils, calcium, iron, Echinacea, garlic pills, vitamins C, D & E and vitamin B12 and all sorts of natural arthritis pain relief tablets. She bought me aids to help me out at home, special bandages, heated cushions and wheat bags, to name just a few. For years, she sent me to acupuncture, reflexology, healing, homeopathy and anything else that she thought might offer a glimmer of hope to make me better. How my parents still had money to pay the bills, I'm not entirely sure.

Both Mum and Aba accompanied me to my first appointment with Dr. Keat. Again, I couldn't make it from the car to the clinic so I was pushed in a wheelchair, which I hated but had to accept as I was too tired to walk – or to argue about it. Dr. Keat's clinic was in a newly built part of the hospital, just down the corridor from the physio and hydro department. The clinic was called 'The Arthritis Centre' and it was almost nice to know there was a clinic dedicated to the disease.

Dr. Keat was like a breath of fresh air. He was a short, middle-aged man, with greying hair and smiling eyes. As I entered the room he shook my hand very firmly which, although Mum always says is a good sign in a man, hurt my fragile hand a little.

We told him everything that had happened and I expressed my concerns over what the M had done to me. He was understanding and sympathetic and reassured me in every way possible. He assured me that I knew my body better than anyone else and that I probably knew arthritis better than any doctor, because I was the one who was feeling it. He was the only doctor in the seventeen years I'd had arthritis to say that to us. He explained how he would continue weaning me off the drug and offered all the other drugs available, including those that were very rarely offered on the NHS as they were so expensive.

I thanked him, but hastily said no to Infliximab and

Sulphasalazine – and anything else that would be infused into my bloodstream. I shuddered at the thought of another drug that might make me feel as if I had cancer. I wanted to get the M out of my system and go back to the old way of doing things – naturally. I was the only one who had treated my arthritis through homeopathy, healing, diet and a whole lot of positive attitude and, lo and behold, I was the only person in my hydro group who didn't look 'arthritic' – again, not a coincidence in my view. I would do it this way again and I would get my body back to the way it once was, if not better. I didn't quite know how just yet, but I knew I'd do it.

I am also sure that were it not for my amazing mum, I would not have had this outlook because, on the days when I couldn't get out of bed, she was the one who pushed me to move. Sometimes she seemed harsh and I felt that she didn't see how much pain I was in, but she did. She would go off and cry afterwards somewhere where I couldn't see her, because it hurt her to push me that much but, deep down, she knew that I had to find strength from somewhere, and she was the only one who could give it to me. Whenever I saw her pushing me or trying hard to help me, I would think about how awful I was to her during previous years and I wished I could rewind the clock and change so many things.

I had three-monthly check-ups with Dr. Keat, who played along with whatever method I wanted to follow to heal myself and, eventually, I weaned myself off the drug. It had done so much damage to me – physically and emotionally. I was exhausted and in constant pain. Everything required too much effort. Even eating was a huge task, as my jaw was so stiff and painful that I could barely chew.

Unfortunately, the drug had also damaged my liver, as I found out later. I was told that I had to be careful and could never drink alcohol again. At this point, I didn't really care. I hadn't had an alcoholic drink for over a year and drinking was the last thing I felt like doing anyway.

I went back to Dr. Graham at St Thomas', who told me that my eye was no better; in fact, the cataract was growing thicker, the pressure had dropped to 3 and there was more inflammation. During that awful year on M, I had become side-tracked with everything else that was going on and, in the end, I forgot the main reason for taking the M. It was, of course, for my eye. I wondered why the hell I had spent a year making myself sick, when I still couldn't have the operation to make me see again.

Dr. Graham was a great doctor and she did everything she could, but she really didn't know what to do after that. I asked her if there were any other ophthalmic doctors who specialised in uveitis and she recommended a doctor at Moorfields Eye Hospital, Mr. Carlos Pavesio, who was known worldwide for his work with uveitis and who had a whole clinic dedicated to the disease.

My parents accompanied me to Moorfields to visit Mr. Pavesio. I couldn't believe that there was this huge hospital dedicated purely to eyes. How many eye problems could there be? When I met Mr. Pavesio, I was completely taken aback. He was handsome, beautifully dressed and softly spoken. I had felt guilty about leaving Dr. Graham after all these years, but now I felt confident and happy with the decision I had made.

Mr. Pavesio was from Brazil and had travelled all over the world giving lectures about uveitis. Something about him made me trust him. He looked at my eye through the slit lamp machine and told us what we knew, that it was very inflamed. He said that, in order to take out this rapidly growing cataract, we had to somehow bring down the inflammation. He suggested that I have another steroid injection in the eye and go from there. Mr. Pavesio, like Dr. Keat, was very kind and understood why I was now even more against conventional medicine than I had been before, but he said that we had to do all we could to get this cataract out. He suggested taking a very short influx of oral steroids along with the steroid injection, to increase the chances of the injection working. I was not at all comfortable with this, but he assured me that I would not get the long-term side effects as I wouldn't be taking it for long enough. Mum, Aba and I took a break to discuss it. Although I was against ever taking any chemical drugs again, I was losing my sight and was running out of options. Mr. Pavesio was only asking me to be on steroids for a month or so to keep the inflammation down. I knew that the worst short-term side effect with steroids was weight gain. Mr. Pavesio said that I would probably have a bigger appetite and my face might swell a little. As Mum and I stood outside the hospital talking it through, I made her promise that if she saw I was eating too much to stop me and if I got too fat to tell me. With everything else going on, the thought of looking like the Michelin Man was enough to send me over the edge.

In the end, I agreed to try the steroids as long as I was monitored carefully, that they would listen if I said I was feeling unwell and that I wouldn't have to be on them for too long. Mr. Pavesio agreed and gave me the drugs, along with the instructions on how to take them, and booked me in for my injection.

I told Lubina what was happening and yet again she co-operated. I carried on having my treatments with her and rationalised it by thinking of Lubina taking care of my joints and Mr. Pavesio fixing my eye.

Aba took me to have my eye injection, as Mum had been taking so much time off work to accompany me to appointments. It was the usual process of putting on the hospital gown and ugly knickers, putting my hair in the hairnet provided and letting the doctor draw a big black arrow on my forehead pointing down to the eye to be injected. I wondered how people who had been to medical school couldn't tell their left from their right? I shivered uncontrollably, as I always did when nervous, as my bed was taken down to the operating theatre and waited for those perfect few moments when the anaesthetic made me feel as if no pain had ever existed. I was home that same evening. I didn't need to stay in overnight any more. My eye was very painful after the injection and I was drowsy after the general anaesthetic, but happy to be going home to sleep in my own bed.

The girls came over the next day as they always did after I'd had an awful day and they piled into my small room, making me laugh as they joked about me looking like a pirate with a patch over my eye. I only had a single bed and a small bedroom, but they didn't care. I'd have three of them on the bed with me, one on my computer chair and two on the floor and I loved it – my very own support network.

Naturally, the steroids showed themselves quicker in me than in other people and my face puffed up like a balloon within three weeks. It was sudden – I only noticed it one day when I glanced in the mirror and my face dropped. "I have a moon face, don't I?" I sulked. I saw Mum's expression – she was waiting for me to explode in self-pity at the thought of looking fat. "It's just a little bit puffy, darling, it's not dreadful," she said gamely. I felt ugly. No clothes looked nice and, anyway, that didn't matter, as I wasn't going out anywhere. I couldn't get around and, even if I could, I didn't want people to see me this way. Mum said that I was mad and that people couldn't see what I was seeing. She assured me that, apart from the short time that the steroids made me puff out a bit, I looked normal and beautiful. Yeah, right. Inflammation is a funny old thing though. There was so much fluid floating around my body that I didn't feel like me. All my joints were swollen and I knew that Mum was lying – people must be able to see what I saw in the mirror: a swollen, ugly crippled girl with a fat face and thinned hair.

A month passed and I started to feel very ill again. The steroids sped up my heart rate and I began to suffer palpitations and panic attacks regularly. That was it for me.

I would give it a go if it meant that I could have the operation but, as the inflammation was not budging, I told Mr. Pavesio I would be weaning myself off the steroids. Along with not being able to walk, eat properly, socialise and see, I didn't want to be a fat person with a heart condition too.

I was being treated homeopathically by Lubina every week, going to the Sanctuary every Sunday and had even started listening to meditation tapes that Jojo had given me. I was trying to keep a positive attitude, but I felt unwell and as if I was running out of options. That's when Mum heard from her friend Tamara in Israel.

Mum now worked as a travel agent for a company that specialised in holidays to Israel and Tamara was based in their Tel Aviv office. Tamara had Crohn's Disease and was so sick at one point that she didn't know if she'd make it to the next day. She had lost so much weight that she could barely move and was on too much medication to mention. Then she found out about Ady Shanan and IPEC Therapy.

Ady had cured her of Crohn's disease through the therapy, which was completely natural and involved no medicine whatsoever, and she was now a healthy woman again. She told Mum that she was sure it could work for me – holistic medicine doesn't just treat one disease. Mum suggested that we go to Israel to meet Ady. We had a family wedding coming up in Tel Aviv, so the timing was perfect. For the first time in what seemed like a very long time, I felt as if there was some hope.

Chapter 8

Back to the Holy Land

Mum and I went out to Israel in August and Tamara picked us up from the airport, slightly shocked to meet me for the first time in a wheelchair. Tamara and her boyfriend lived on a Moshav in Israel just outside Tel Aviv. A Moshav is like a small village or settlement, where each family has a private house and some land and there is usually a farm involved. The houses are usually passed down through generations, so the current residents are more willing to keep up the beauty. Tamara's Moshav was out of this world. Her house itself was beautiful; all on one level with a huge furnace-style fireplace in the middle of the lounge (it was never really cold enough in Israel to use it, except for maybe a month or two in the winter, but Tamara loved the style of it), a gorgeous outdoor breakfast area just off the huge kitchen and the garden was magnificent. There was a seating area on the patio and their garden led into the fields behind. At sunset and sunrise it was just magical. On our first night, we sat there after dinner, watching the sun go down and for the first time in ages I felt at peace.

We stayed at Tamara's for two days. During this time she took us to some fabulous places where I'd never been before, including an Arab hummus restaurant in Jaffa serving only hummus and pitta. Then she showed us the flea market, which was also quite extraordinary. There was a little café in the depths of the flea market that, in a way, reminded me of an English tea house. Everything in the café was up for sale. Every chair, every tea cup and every picture on the wall. It was an experience. We sat at a table outside drinking mint tea and my body enjoyed being bathed by the hot sun.

After our short stay with Tamara, we went to Netanya for the remainder of the holiday and stayed in a family-run hotel owned by a good friend of Aba. It was nice to have some time alone with Mum, relaxing on the beach, going for lunch and sitting around Netanya Square with nowhere really to go. We also spent a lot of time with the family, especially Uncle Asher and Aunty Zahava, the ones who threw the infamous parties when we were kids and whose kids were now all grown up. Their eldest, Keren offered to drive us to meet Ady Shanan.

It took us about an hour to get to Givat-Ada, which was a stunning little village with vineyards and orchards in every direction I looked. The drive up there made me realise that there was so much of Israel I hadn't yet seen, so many beautiful places. Ady's wife opened the door to greet us and, as we walked into the house, Ady walked towards us. He was tall, handsome and polite. Although I was fluent in Hebrew, he spoke to me in English, as he knew that it would be easier for me to both explain my situation and understand his description of IPEC in that language.

Although he had a treatment room at the back of his house, his clinic was in Ramat Aviv, a northern neighbourhood of Tel Aviv. He explained about IPEC. IPEC stands for Integrated Physical Emotional Clearing and, although its name has since been changed to BAMIA for legal reasons, I will refer to it here as IPEC as that is what it was called when I was in treatment. It is recent, developed since 1997, and is only available in Israel and in parts of North

America. It is based on an integration of many principles from the fields of oriental medicine (acupuncture), psychology, kinesiology, bioenergy, Kabbalah, homeopathy and chiropractic, to name a few. It can treat many illnesses, be they physical, mental, emotional or spiritual. Special tools are used that measure the energy flow in your body, your Chi, the life energy that the Chinese discovered thousands of years ago and that circulates via energy pathways through all parts of the body. This subtle energy is constantly flowing throughout our bodies, via the Meridian system, to the organs, tissues and cells.

IPEC believes that any blockage, misdirection or other disruption in the flow and balance of the Chi can result in pain, dysfunction or ill health. Our physical and mental health is strongly affected by this energy flow and, in order to fix an illness, the Chi must be unblocked.

Ady explained that he would ask my body questions through a technique called Muscle Testing, or Applied Kinesiology. It sounds so strange and, believe me, I didn't know how to react to it myself at first, but it works like this: I would sit on the edge of the treatment bed, hold my right arm up in front of me and Ady would put two fingers on my forearm. I was told to hold my arm up against his fingers and stop them from pushing my arm down. When he asked, 'is your name Lauren?' my arm stayed in place. When he then asked 'Is your name Lisa?' without any choice at all my arm fell down to my lap and I had no control over it. I couldn't hold my arm up. This was muscle testing, asking my subconscious mind a question and it responding by saying 'yes' or 'no' – strong or weak. If 'yes', my arm would stay up and if 'no', my arm would drop. This is how Ady would get my subconscious to tell him what he needed to know in order to be able to use the right techniques and help me get better. This way he would get the information he needed to diagnose me and then he would ask what to do - how he could re-programme my body so that its energy blocks would disappear and not come back.

Ady told me that the clearing process is carried out through a variety of interventions using the Meridian system and other reflex points in the body. It wasn't an easy process to understand but over time I started to understand it a bit more. After someone has had an illness for a long time, the body sees anything that comes its way as potentially dangerous, so it tries to fight it off. It does this by throwing out an allergic reaction. The allergic reaction does not necessarily mean sneezing and a runny nose; it could be a flare-up of the arthritis. In the past few years, the doctors had told me to stop eating wheat, dairy, sugar and acidic foods, amongst others. What Ady wanted to do was to work these 'allergies' out of my system, so that my body could accept anything. It made sense. He would unblock my Chi to make my body healthy again and bring these so called 'allergies' out of my system, allowing me to stay healthy and not flare up every time I ate, drank or touched something that my body saw as dangerous.

He told me about people with various physical and mental illnesses who had been cured by IPEC and I believed him, because of Tamara. Also, there was a truth about him that made me trust and believe in him.

After discussing my particular problem, Ady was sure that he could help me, but I would have to be around for about three months. I thanked him and told him that I would discuss it with my family and we would let him know. If we took into account how much it would cost for me to stay in Israel for so long, plus the cost of the treatment itself, it would come to about £3,000. We went back to Netanya and discussed it at length and we also phoned Aba to talk to him about it. Apart from the fact that we didn't have £3,000, I didn't have anywhere to stay either. We didn't have our own place in Israel and, although we stayed with family when we went for holidays, no one likes to outstay their welcome.

The next day, Mum's friend Solange came from Jerusalem to see us. She arrived at our hotel very early and I woke up in excruciating pain. I could barely move my legs or use my hands and I couldn't open my jaw at all. I was crying but the more I cried the more my jaw hurt because of the pressure. Mum and Solange didn't know what to do. They went downstairs to get me some breakfast, thinking that maybe eating would loosen my jaw. When they brought the food up to the room, I could see that they had both been crying which made me even more upset. I didn't want people to be upset because of me. Mum tried feeding me a yoghurt, but I couldn't open my mouth enough to get the spoon inside and it hurt too much to try, so I managed to swallow some painkillers with water through a straw and tried to go back to sleep.

Later on that day, Aba rang to tell us that Uncle Asher had offered to let me stay with them for however long I needed to finish the treatment. He would be pleased, he said, as having had five children and only two now living at home, there was plenty of room and it would be nice for my cousin, Moran, who was only a year younger than me.

The next day I was feeling a little better, so we went round to Uncle Asher and Aunty Zahava to thank them.

Back in London, I could only think about one thing. I had a feeling that this treatment would change my life and I really wanted to give it a go, but money was an issue. Money had proved to be another problem with which April from the hospital had helped me. Mum and I had been discussing the difficulties of finding and keeping jobs with April and her mum in the waiting room one day. April had tried to work and had had a few jobs in the past but found it too hard to stand all day when she worked in a bakery, and too hard to sit all day in an office. I had aspirations though and didn't want to work in a shop or a bakery and I certainly didn't want to do a mundane job that would be 'suitable' for me because I was considered disabled. I told April that I hated never having any money of my own and always having to rely on my parents. She asked if I received Disability Living Allowance. I had never heard of it. She said it was available if you were disabled and needed help with money and getting around. We looked into it and Mum became furious – why had no one told us about this before? This money is awarded to the parents of a disabled child until the child reaches the age of sixteen. With all the time Mum and Aba had taken off work and the number of hospital trips that we had made, a bit of extra money would have come in very handy. They had had to spend out on special shoes, equipment, homeopathy and so much more. Why did our GP or any of the doctors never tell us about it?

After we got in touch with the Department for Work and Pensions, they carried out an evaluation. They could clearly see that I was unable to move, so they awarded me the middle rate, which basically meant I would get about £200 a month. It wasn't a lot, but it would certainly help. I was still angry that I had had arthritis for seventeen years and no one had ever told us that we could get help.

This £200 a month, however, would not pay for my treatment in Israel. My parents wanted me to have the treatment, as we all believed it could help, so they took out a loan. Along with the millions of things they have done for me over the years, this is something I will always appreciate and never forget. We called Ady to tell him I'd be coming at the beginning of November, after my cousin's London wedding in October, and we confirmed with my uncle and aunt that they were still happy for me to stay with them in Israel.

I went to say goodbye to everyone before I left. I thanked Andre at my final physio session and, as always, he was very supportive. Dr. Keat wished me the best of luck and told me to contact him when I returned. Mr. Pavesio seemed slightly pessimistic, but said that he really hoped that the treatment worked and that hopefully in a few months from now we could operate on the eye. Lubina, of course, was as understanding as ever. She said that she knew about muscle testing and could do it herself. It reassured me to know that this was a real method that Lubina had learned too.

On the Saturday before I left, the girls and I arranged a big night out to say goodbye. Natalie, Zoe and I shopped in Oxford Street during the day and, as we sat down over coffee, we spoke about shopping when I came back from Israel. I said that the next time I went shopping with them I would be able to walk around the shops for hours on end and not get tired and not be in pain. I was determined to make this happen. I had really started to acquire a taste for fashion and loved shopping, but didn't have the energy (or the money) to do it too often.

That night Zoe and I got ready at Natalie's house. I was determined to get dolled up and make myself look gorgeous and, somehow, I squeezed myself into a pair of heels and got on with it. The girls insisted that we stop by my house to drop off my stuff, telling me that it would be easier than leaving it in the car. I found it a bit odd but didn't question it. When I walked into my house, I was greeted with a very loud 'SURPRISE!' from my friends and family who were all there for my surprise leaving party. I was so shocked that I didn't know what to do and when I saw Nanny standing at the back of the lounge looking so old and frail, I walked over to her and began to cry.

It was a lovely evening and I was able to say goodbye to everyone properly. The girls gave me a huge card and present and it was a perfect way to spend my last day with them.

Two days later I was in Israel. Aba came with me to get me settled in and Aunty Zahava had made Keren's old room into my new room with a double bed, a TV, two empty wardrobes and a dressing table. I took photo frames and albums with me and put them up all over my room.

Aba joined me for my first session with Ady and we got to see his amazing clinic for the first time. It was within a country club in Ramat Aviv, about twenty minutes from Netanya. Again, Ady started with the very bizarre muscle testing technique and Aba was fascinated.

As the sessions went on, Ady stopped asking the questions out loud and just mumbled them to himself to save time. He still got accurate answers though. He showed me a box full of tiny little labelled bottles, in which were the components of different things, such as wheat, dairy, sugar, citrus fruits, salt and even things as simple as oxygen, metal and wood. Every session he would ask my body what it wanted to work on. If, for example, it said 'wheat', I would hold the bottle with the wheat component in one hand, choose at random three crystals from a big box and hold them in the other hand, while Ady used a very strange instrument to tap from the crown of my head all the way down to the bottom of my back. The crystals would take the negative energy of the wheat out of my body and put positive energy back in and the tapping device somehow helped this. I don't know how this worked and I still don't understand it fully, but what I do know is that I arrived at the airport in Israel in a wheelchair and, within three weeks of seeing Ady, I was riding a bike, something I hadn't been able to do for many years.

Ady made me see life in a different way. He brought positivity back into my life and showed me how important positivity is for a person and how badly negative energies can affect one's life. It all made so much sense and I realised how my own mind probably had more to do with my ill health than I had ever thought. I had a great deal of pent-up anger and frustration within me and there were many things that I still hadn't dealt with, but Ady made me understand how important energies are and it forced me to deal with my anger. Ady had a very calming effect on me and I'm sure I am not the only one who felt it. I could be really angry or upset at the start of a session but, as soon as he walked into the room, things didn't seem so bad and I would relax straight away.

One treatment always differed slightly from the one before, but they were pretty much the same. After the treatment, I had to stay in the room on my own for anything up to an hour and meditate. I had started doing this at home with Jojo's tapes, so I had learnt the basics and Ady taught me the rest, including how to find my centre and how to relax, but basically meditation is an individual thing and you do what is best for your body and mind. After the treatment, I couldn't touch what we had worked on for twenty-four hours. For instance, after the wheat treatment I couldn't have any wheat for twenty-four hours and after that my body would be able to accept it. The one instance that I found the funniest was when we worked on metal and I couldn't touch anything metal for twenty-four hours. This was hard as I couldn't open doors or use cutlery. I arrived at my Aunt's house for lunch and had to walk up the stairs to the eighth floor apartment, as I couldn't use the lift.

Just as well that I could now walk again!

I was usually very tired after my treatment sessions, so I would go to my Aunt Gila, have lunch with her and the girls and then sleep there for a short while. Uncle Asher's house was big but often empty, as he and my aunt were out at work and Moran was in the army and, as I found it rather cold and lonely sometimes, I preferred to be with Gila who, like myself, liked everything to be clean and tidy. I felt at home with her because she reminded me so much of Mum. She was always cleaning and cooking and fussing over the kids. I could also talk to her about anything and she became a second mother to me while I was in Israel.

My cousin Anat had moved to Israel from South Africa at the same time as me to join the Israeli army for two years. Her family had an apartment in the centre of Netanya and, when she was home from her army base, she would usually be alone there. Moran and I spent a lot of time with her and the three of us became like sisters. I had also made contact with some friends I had known from my childhood and, luckily, I managed to make some good friends and enjoy a social life while I was there. I went out with friends and cousins in Tel Aviv; I often sat having coffee or dinner in Netanya Square with Anat and rode my bike along the promenade every day. With every session I had with Ady, I felt better and better. I started to change the way I thought about things. It became apparent that if my subconscious had done all this work, then it really is true that everything starts in the mind and the power of the mind can heal anything.

I meditated daily and started to be able to shut off completely. I got to the point of being able to block out every noise from the outside world. It was November, so the weather was temperamental when I first got there, but there were some days when it was sunny and warm enough to sit on the beach meditating. I did this as often as I could and also started visualisation exercises. I would sit on the sand, in front of the sea, listening to the waves crashing on the shore and visualised myself being healthy, doing all the things I wanted to do, from simple things like walking around with loads of shopping bags on my arms, to acting in a TV programme or film. While meditating on the beach, I remembered how I used to feel in hydro sessions, seeing the picture of the dolphins in the sea when I was stuck in the hot, sweaty hydro pool, feeling the humidity and condensation all over my body. I wanted to be cool and free like the dolphins. I now felt that I was.

I spent a lot of time with Tamara in her Moshav or in the flea market in Jaffa and I also learned how to cook with Gila. Gila taught me our family's favourite Moroccan dishes and I picked it up quite quickly.

One day, when we were making some cakes for a family party, Mum called with some bad news. Nanny had been having tests done and the results showed that she had liver cancer. I started crying on the phone and felt helpless and far away. I wanted to be there for her, but Mum insisted that Nanny wanted me to get better more than anything and that I should finish the treatment before I came home.

Every time I spoke to Mum, she seemed so sad. She was leaving work in her lunch hour to see Nanny, then back to work, then to Nanny again after work and, at the weekends, Nanny was with Mum at our house. Mum was exhausted and sad at the same time. Eventually Nanny moved into our house and into my room, as I wasn't there, and so she didn't feel that she was such a burden, something she always felt even though the family preferred to have her there so that they knew she was all right. Mum arranged a carer to come for Nanny and she came daily, arriving before Mum left for work and leaving when Aba got home, so there was always someone with Nanny. That comforted me, but I still felt helpless.

Very early one morning in late January, I was woken up by someone getting into bed with me. I thought I was dreaming but I wasn't – it was Mum! She had come to surprise me. I was so happy to see her and I moved into her hotel with her for the week, the same hotel we had been in only five months earlier when I couldn't move my hands, legs or jaw. Now I was a different person. Mum couldn't believe the change in me and she was so excited about it but she had one thing on her mind all the time and that was Nanny. She told me that she and Nanny had spoken a lot about the cancer and about her fate and they had cried, laughed, joked and had come to accept it. I always felt that being a very spiritual family has helped us to understand and accept death and illnesses, but it was still difficult. The week passed and Mum went home but her visit gave me even more strength and determination to get completely better. I wanted to arrive back in London unrecognisable to everyone. I wanted them to see that I was able-bodied and rejuvenated.

I wouldn't know how my eye was doing until I saw Mr. Pavesio, but Ady and I worked on visualisation techniques to try to help. I think I focused too much on the arthritis side of things and not enough on the eye, but I just wanted to walk, eat and use my hands properly again.

After three and a half months, I can honestly say I was exactly how I had visualised myself. I was healthy, able-bodied, rejuvenated and happy. I was ready to start my life again. I had also decided to give acting another go, but I wanted to study interior design. I don't know where the idea came from – it just came to me one day and I wondered why I had never thought about it before. I had always been fascinated by houses and wanted to know what the inside of other people's houses looked like.

I was constantly re-arranging furniture at home when I was young and would get into trouble for moving stuff around. I wasn't great with sewing, or physically making things, but I had great ideas and everyone always said I had an eye for detail. I always knew I wanted to work within a creative field and too much time had passed to be able to go to uni and do my directing degree. It was sad, after having made so many plans but time had passed and life had changed. I needed to get back and start earning money. I needed to contribute and help my parents after all the money they'd spent on me so I needed to figure out how I could do what I enjoyed while still earning money.

Ady had warned me that IPEC needed 'maintenance' treatments every few months to keep it working, otherwise eventually the body could revert back to how it was. There was no way I could stay in Israel forever, but I felt fantastic now and was sure that I could keep myself like this and see Ady whenever I went back to Israel to visit.

Whatever was going to happen to me in the future, Ady had taught me the most important lesson, a lesson that would get me through anything that was thrown at me. He made me realise that I *could* get better. It didn't matter how sick I was; it was never the end. As long as I believed that I could get better, I always would. So, now the trick was to believe that I was healthy - and then I would stay healthy. There is no tool more powerful than the mind.

I stayed in Israel for a total of five months and came back to London a week after having celebrated my twentieth birthday with friends and family in a karaoke bar in Netanya.

Chapter 9

Burning the Candle

Mum, Aba and Ilana came to the airport and Nanny was waiting at home with her carer. She was so frail and little but she was so happy to see me. She was still living with us and staying in my room, so I slept on the couch most nights unless Ilana agreed to swap with me.

It was great to see the girls again and, thankfully, it was as if nothing had changed. We were just as close as we had always been and now I was now able to enjoy life with them in a way I never had before; untainted by disability, drugs and depression.

I had found an interior design course at a local private college that started in September, so I landed a job in the meantime as a fashion merchandiser for a company that manufactured clothes in Hong Kong and supplied them to the major fashion retail stores. Mum helped me find the job, as her friend, Martin, ran the company. I was due to start on 19th April.

That morning, we awoke to a nightmare. Nanny had had a heart attack. We called an ambulance and Mum and Aba planned to follow it to the hospital. Mum told me that I should go to work on my first day. I protested, saying that I wanted to be with Nanny, but she insisted and promised to call me if

Nanny took a turn for the worse. Reluctantly, I went. Getting a job like this was a big deal for me. Being able to work at all was a big deal, but I knew that being there while Nanny was in hospital would make me distant and unfocused and I didn't want that. More than that, I wanted to be with Nanny. My colleagues were lovely and it was a great company, but the day dragged and I could only focus on one thing. Eventually, the day ended and I went straight to the hospital.

When I arrived, Nanny looked lifeless. Her mouth was open and I wet her lips with cotton buds to try to make her more comfortable. The whole family had arrived, including Uncle Harry, Aunty Ruth and my cousins, Stacey and Mark. Ilana was there too. The eight of us surrounded her bed and, when Mum asked if she wanted anything, she replied – completely out of character – "a pound out the till." It was a phrase that only Poppa would have said, and we decided that he must've been standing there with us, waiting for her. We could imagine him standing next to the bed saying in his best East End accent, 'What d'they think you bleedin' want? Tell 'em a pound out the till.' Apparently, this was an East End Cockney saying. A few seconds after that remark, the beeps on her heart monitor started to get closer and closer together, until it was one long beep, and we knew she was gone. The doctors came in and everyone left the cubicle – except me. I hugged her and couldn't bring myself to stop, because I knew I would never get to hug my amazing nanny again. Natalie and Zoe turned up and tried to help me to leave, but I screamed at everyone to leave me there for a while. Eventually, they led me to the room where everyone else was waiting.

I was absolutely devastated and Mum was inconsolable. I sat on the floor in the corridor with Natalie and Zoe, just crying and talking. They called our other friends, including Simi, who was at university in Brighton. At midnight that same night, Simi got on a train to London so that she would be with me the next day. There are not many people who would be that selfless and over time most of my friendships have changed along the way but Simi has always been the one constant in my life, the one who would get on a train at midnight regardless of what she had going on, just to be with me. Simi and I were always so different, but our friendship only ever strengthened over the years.

That night, we thought that it would be too late to organise the funeral for the following day, Tuesday, but as it was Mum's birthday on the Wednesday, she really wanted to do everything she could to hold it on the Tuesday, to stop all her future birthdays being tainted; associated with the day she buried her mother. Luckily, we were able to arrange it for the next day. So many people came to pay their respects and it made me realise how loved my Nanny had been. She died exactly a month after I returned from Israel and I know that she waited for me to get better before she left us. It really comforts me to know that she got to see me so healthy.

In the Jewish religion, when someone dies, the immediate family have to 'sit shiva', which means they sit on low chairs while the Rabbi says prayers every night for seven days and friends and family come to watch them mourn. The shiva took place at our house which was a good thing because there were always people around to distract us from our sadness but when it was over the house was eerily quiet.

I refused to go into my room for over a week after Nanny died, as it reminded me too much of her but eventually life started going back to normal. I took and passed my driving test on May 26th 2004. I had previously taken two tests before moving to Israel, but wasn't ready for the first one and, during the second, I was in too much pain to drive properly. Things had changed now and passing my driving test was just the next stage in gaining back my independence. I still had the money saved from the New Year's Eve car accident I'd had with Natalie a few years before and I managed to buy myself an old Peugeot 306 with the money. It was blue or green, depending on the light, and I loved it.

I had a new-found freedom and independence that I'd never before experienced. The car, the job, the income, the social life – I felt like a grown-up; a healthy, arthritis-free grown-up.

Although some would have found mine a dream job, it wasn't for me. I had only just started living life again and felt as if I could do anything. Acting was always in the back of my mind, I still dreamed about being an actress and wished I'd get the opportunity to make a film, or even a TV show, and I wanted to be on stage and I still slightly resented the fact that I missed out on my university years. I was also excited about starting my interior design course – my back-up plan to acting but still something that I'd always wanted to do. My mind just wasn't focused on the job I was in. I wanted to go out and meet new people, to go to random places that I'd never been before and wanted to be spontaneous – just because I could. I didn't last my three-month probation period, but I didn't really care. I knew this was because I wasn't focused enough and they needed someone who was.

I had a great summer swimming, partying and enjoying myself and I was ready to start my course in September. I joined the acting agency that Lana was signed up with and, because my course was only a few days a week, I got a few acting jobs to fill in the other days. Lana and I were put on loads of jobs together, which made it even better. We landed walk-on roles on films starring, amongst others, Jennifer Aniston, Clive Owen, Michelle Pfieffer, Brittany Murphy and Catherine Tate. I had one line (which subsequently never made the final cut) in The Da Vinci Code and I nearly fainted when I met Tom Hanks and Ron Howard. I also had small parts in a few TV shows, such as The Bill and The IT Crowd and did some theatre shows too.

I loved the buzz of the set and the feeling of being on stage was electric. During my time at Performing Arts College, I had got a taste for reading plays and so I spent time reading Shakespeare and Arthur Miller. Lana thought that I was mad as she hated reading plays – and theatre generally – but I loved them both.

In September, I began studying Advanced Interior Design at Oaklands College and turned up with the equipment we had been told to buy to help with the course. As it was only a one-year course, it was very intense and they packed a great deal of information into this short time. I enjoyed every minute of it, especially the hands-on projects. We were given case studies and had to design specific rooms, by making a portfolio of hand-drawn floor plans, elevations and instructions to trade, as well as providing work and cost schedules, furniture plans, colour charts and mood boards. It was a lot of work but I loved every minute, I loved being able to be openly creative. I would sit in the lounge for hours on end, slowly drawing and painting my room designs and Mum would always comment on my patience. For some reason, I seemed to be patient only with animals, elderly people and art. I suppose that with art, I was able to completely immerse myself in what I was doing and forget about everything else.

Dave and I also solidified our friendship during this time and started spending more time together. I'd missed him and realised how close we were, like brother and sister. My mum said he spent more time at our house than Ilana.

My social life was also back on track. I began to do club promotions with a friend, Katie, and a group of promoters who held club nights in a few London clubs. We worked for them at least two nights a week, if not more, for a bit of extra cash and I couldn't believe the turn my life had taken. Last year I hadn't even been able to go out with my friends for dinner and now, a year later, I was working in clubs. Sometimes we would be the door girls – seeing who could come in and who couldn't – or we would work on the till taking the entrance fees and, at other times, we helped out inside the club, especially when there were live acts performing. These were the best nights, not only because so many people turned up but also because we showcased some of the best talent on the UK music scene, as well as some US artists, and we went up on stage with them and partied afterwards in the VIP section.

After a few months, Katie and I started working for other promotion companies, companies that held larger, more high-profile events, such as award show after-parties and birthday celebrations for footballers, actors and singers. At first, it was amazing, as we met some really interesting people and loved the buzz that surrounded these celebrities, but their pretentiousness wore thin after a while. They were fun to be around at the beginning but the way they acted got boring. We saw footballers cheating on their wives and girlfriends, reality TV stars getting drunker than could ever be imagined and actors and socialites snorting lines of cocaine on the tables in the VIP area. It didn't faze us, this was just part and parcel of the London club scene.

Aside from the pretentiousness of the London party scene, we had the most incredible time. Most of my friends were starting to settle into jobs and, I suppose, grow up. But Katie loved going out – weekends, weekdays, she didn't care – and that suited me because I wanted to make the most of being young and healthy. I did my utmost to forget about what it felt like to have arthritis. I stopped meditating, doing Pilates and all the positive thinking exercises that Ady had taught me. I wasn't going to the Sanctuary anymore and I didn't even start seeing Lubina again. I was living for the now and that was all that mattered. I had big dreams and I didn't want even the thought of arthritis coming back into my head and ruining them again.

Natalie and her family moved out of the area and, although we were all still friendly, things changed when she started going out with Darren.

Everyone except Zoe noticed a change in her, mainly because Zoe's boyfriend was friendly with Natalie's and so they still saw a lot of each other. The rest of us who were single, however, took a back seat in Natalie's new life. Darren was textbook perfect for her – a Jewish doctor who was a few years older than her, with good prospects and a good family – a far cry from Jake and the life that Natalie didn't care to remember anymore.

The way I saw it was that we did go through all the things we went through all those years ago, and that couldn't be changed. All we could do was accept that that period in time did, in fact, happen, learn from the mistakes, and move on. Natalie didn't want to acknowledge that part of her life anymore – and I was a big part of that life. All she had ever really wanted was to get married and have children, so when she met the man who could give that to her, she didn't want to ruin her chances by having a person around who might spill the beans on certain aspects of her past that she didn't want him knowing.

As the months went on, she pushed me further and further away and it hurt. She was my one of my best friends; we had gone through so much together and yet she was willing to throw it all away because she was in a relationship. Even when I was living in Israel, she would be the one person who would text me every day without fail telling me how much she missed me and what was going on in her life and this was all changing so quickly. She began to only go out with Darren, his friends and their partners.

In March, my 21st birthday coincided with Mum's 50th and my parents' 25th wedding anniversary so Mum and Aba decided to hold a big party for all our friends and family. I am telling you, there are people who don't hold weddings as big as this party! We held it in the really beautiful Regency Banqueting Suite in Finchley. Aba's friend Ami, who owned an Israeli restaurant in Golders Green, provided the food. The hall was owned by Ami's brother and the entertainment and music was provided by a friend of the family. Two hundred guests were invited.

Uncle Asher and Aunty Zahava came over from Israel, along with other family members from Israel, South Africa and Paris. A few of us gave speeches and Mum and Aba presented me with the most wonderful present – they had named a star after me. It was the most fantastic evening and we ate, drank and danced to Israeli and English music. Dave was my substitute boyfriend for the night and he fitted the role perfectly, by turning up in a beautiful suit, sitting next to me at dinner and dancing with me.

Natalie and Darren had been invited to the party but, after that, Natalie and I barely spoke and when we did speak, we argued. The more I tried to talk to her about the situation, to make her understand that I was upset, the more she pushed me away. She claimed that I was jealous of her relationship and wanted to sabotage it, which was ridiculous. More than anything, I wanted her to be happy – I just wanted to be able to share that happiness with her.

Eventually, I tired of her arguing with me and accusing me of jealousy and so we just stopped speaking.

It was hard for me to come to terms with, because we had been through so much together and she knew things about me that no one knew – and vice versa. I heard once that friends are there for a reason, a season or a lifetime, and I guess that Natalie was there for a season, or perhaps even a reason, when I needed her, but when it came to real friendship, she wasn't really the friend that I had hoped she was, or the friend that I was to her.

I had started working on the final project for my interior design course and became really involved in it – I really wanted to get good grades and I believed I could. What with the course, the acting jobs and the club promotions, I was kept busy most of the time, and I was grateful for that.

Dr. Keat was happy with my drastic improvement and, although none of the doctors wanted to admit that an alternative treatment had worked better than their methods, I was living proof and Dr. Keat could see this. One of my check-ups took place on quite a warm summer's day and I arrived wearing a denim mini-skirt. Dr. Keat said that it was fantastic that I could now wear short skirts and feel comfortable in them. "You just keep on doing whatever it is that means you can wear mini-skirts," he said. I laughed, noticing that I was actually the only person in the Arthritis Centre wearing a mini-skirt, or indeed anything that left the joints visible.

Then, out of nowhere, as is always the case, everything changed once again. Although the sight in my right eye had been all but gone for a while, it was now getting worse, much worse. There was not much sight left at all and the eye felt aggravated and sometimes sore. It didn't matter how many drops I put in, this eye just kept getting worse. Mr. Pavesio wasn't as enthusiastic as Dr. Keat. His job was to get my eye healthy again and, as far as he could see, it had only grown worse over the past year. Although he was quite skeptical about alternative treatments, the thing I liked about Mr. Pavesio is that there was a great deal of sincerity to him. When he spoke about not knowing what to do with the predicament we faced, he spoke with passion, as if he genuinely cared what happened to my eye, and my experiences with doctors haven't always been like that. He never rushed me because there were other patients to be seen and he always put a lot of time and thought into what we would do.

He looked in my eye, sat back and gave us the shocking news that there was nothing else that could be done. I was eventually going to totally lose the sight in my right eye. If they removed the cataract while the inflammation was so radically high, there was a 90% chance that I would lose the sight completely anyway and so he said that they were not going to take the chance on the operation as it was so dangerous and other complications could arise. Aba, who had accompanied me to all my Moorfields appointments, began to sob. I didn't know what to feel. The only time I had ever seen him cry was when Safta died, so my initial reaction was to try to comfort him but, at the same time, I had so many other thoughts floating around in my head. I gave him a hug and told him it would be OK. Aba apologised to Mr. Pavesio, but he could not stop crying. Mr. Pavesio understood and I could see that he was upset and frustrated that there was nothing he could do.

When I went home that evening, I shut myself in my room. No matter what had happened to me in the past, I had always believed that I would come through it. I believed that I would come through the worst of the arthritis and, up until this point, I had – and I had never worried too much about my eye for some reason. I suppose that I had always trusted that it would fix itself. But, it wasn't going to fix itself and I was going to be blind in one eye.

I went into Mum's and Aba's room and found our old photo albums. For some reason, I wanted to look through old memories. I sat on their bed with the door closed, crying as I looked through the albums. I refused to speak to anyone, but Mum must have called one of the girls, because later on that evening they predictably showed up and, of course, piled into the room, armed with a human-sized teddy bear and card of the same proportions. Although I was appreciative of their support, there was no cheering me up. I had to come to terms with what I was losing and I could only do that by allowing myself to be upset.

A few days later, I came to the realisation that this was only one eye – I had another one and that worked just fine. I had overcome worse than this and so I would overcome this too.

Apparently, I was going to have more to overcome. Before my final interior design examination, I noticed sporadic pains in my knees, which then spread to my hands, ankles and jaw and I realised that, only ten months after completing my IPEC Therapy, the arthritis had come back. Ady had been right: I needed maintenance treatments to keep my body clean and I wasn't helping myself by burning the candle at both ends. I had spent ten months partying, studying, working, getting up early, going to bed late – and all this with no homeopathy, no meditation or Pilates, or any form of exercise – and my eating habits weren't great either. The stress of finding out about my eye was probably the straw that broke the camel's back.

Chapter 10

Finding the 'Friend'

Though my pains had come back and I had to live with losing the sight in my eye, I still worked really hard at my exams and put every possible bit of effort into my final portfolio. I wasn't going to let this relapse get the better of me. Thankfully, I passed my course and my tutor said that I would make a great interior designer. But I couldn't escape the fact that my joints were getting worse and worse as the days went on and it felt like I'd taken one step forward and twenty steps back.

My knees had swollen up and filled with fluid, my ankles were stiff, my jaw was stiff and painful, my hands and fingers were swollen and I was back in weekly physio and hydro. I had never suffered that badly with my hands before and had always liked my hands – I thought they were quite feminine – but now the ring that my parents had made for me out of the diamonds that Nanny had left me didn't fit on my finger anymore. So I was back to square one and had to look forward to yet another summer in pain. But no, I wasn't going to let myself go back to being that disabled girl that I once was, and neither was Mum.

Dr. Keat referred me to the hand therapy clinic and Aba waited outside while I had my first appointment. All the therapists in this clinic were women and they wore dark green uniforms. My therapist was Karina – a pretty but boyish girl from New Zealand. She sat me down at a table and started talking to me about my hands. I couldn't concentrate on what she was saying, because I was distracted by the strange plastic 'hands' stuck all over the walls. "It looks like Freddie Krueger threw up in here," I remarked to Karina. "They're splints," she told me. "They're to keep your hands from becoming deformed." Well, anything to keep my hands from looking deformed. Karina checked over my hands and told me that the hyper-mobility of my joints was not doing the inflammation any good. The fact that my thumbs could literally move in any direction, with no limit, would increase the inflammation. Karina told me that I would need a few different splints. I remember hearing about splints when I was younger, but Mum had never wanted me to have them as they seemed too severe. Now I understood the need for them, and Mum's reasoning for keeping me away from them.

Karina drew around my hand with a pencil and tissue paper and from that she created the splint by melting flesh-coloured plastic in a huge pot and adding Velcro. It was a pretty clever process, actually. The first splint she made was for my ridiculously opposable thumbs. She said that the more freely they moved, the more the synovial fluid would build up and the joint would in turn become more inflamed. The splint would inhibit the movement to prevent this happening and would also keep the joints in the right place to stop them becoming deformed.

After the splint-making, Karina showed me around the rest of the clinic, which was like a mock house. There were different household items, including kettles, cutlery, showers and toilets, and she assessed how well I managed with each of these. Her evaluation led her to give me a leaflet on disability aids, so I'm guessing that she didn't think I was too capable. She gave my hands a paraffin wax treatment, which was soothing and relaxing. I left the clinic with six splints, a disability aids booklet and information on how to buy a paraffin wax pot. Of course, Mum ordered me one straightaway. Two of the splints were for me to wear at night and they covered my entire hands, all the way up to my elbows. They were ugly and uncomfortable and Karina had warned me that they would hurt at first, as they were putting my hands back in the right positions and it would feel unnatural.

I couldn't sleep properly with the splints as they hurt my hands and every time I turned over I would hit my face with one of them. As soon as I woke up, I would try to hide them in the dedicated plastic box under my bed, but moving and reaching first thing in the morning was not really feasible.

We were back to the days when getting out of bed seemed insurmountable. But Mum pushed me to my limits and made me move. She wouldn't let me end up like some of the girls we knew from physio.

I didn't have the option of going back to Ady because there was not enough money and I would have had to keep going back, or move there permanently, and if I wanted to pursue careers in acting or interior design, London was the place to be. And regardless, I needed to figure out how to keep myself healthy without relying on one, particularly inaccessible treatment. If I wanted to get better, I would have to do it myself. I had to find the will to get better again. I forced myself every day to remember the lessons Ady had taught me, and others I had learned along the way, as well as new things I had yet to learn.

I am the master of my mind. There is no tool more powerful than my mind. If I believe I am healthy, I will be healthy. I think, therefore I am. But it was more than that, my body needed more and I needed to find out what it was.

My anger was still quite prominent, and it was worse during a flare-up as I was extremely temperamental. I took it out on Ilana a lot, mostly because, out of everyone, she seemed like she really didn't get it, or didn't care. I was jealous of her getting ready to go out to parties while I was stuck in bed not able to do anything. Usually the centre of everything, she was not at all shy and could make friends with anyone. One evening, she was in her room with her door open, doing her make-up in preparation for an evening out, and my remote control dropped down the side of my bed. I couldn't reach it myself, so I asked Ilana if she could pick it up for me. "I'm getting ready, Lauren, I don't have time," she replied. I shouted at her, pointing out that it wouldn't take a minute for her to pick it up, but she refused. I went absolutely mad, screaming, shouting and swearing. She was able to go out and I was stuck in bed, again, but she couldn't even do one small thing for me because it took up too much of her precious getting-ready time. I was furious and as the days went on I just couldn't let the matter drop. That night I had to wait 45 minutes until someone came upstairs so that I could turn on my TV. It may not seem like a big deal, but when you're lying in bed with nothing else to do, the TV keeps you company – I couldn't even hold a book because my hands hurt so much. More than that, I couldn't understand how Ilana could be so unhelpful when it made no difference to her to pick up my remote control for me. I couldn't let it go.

A few days later, it was Saturday morning and I had made it down to the lounge to sit on the couch. Ilana was sitting on the armchair and I shouted at her with attitude to change the channel. She shouted back, saying that she would watch what she wanted to watch and that was it. This resulted in me confronting her about the remote control situation and it turned into the screaming match that had been brewing.

She accused me of being spoilt and expecting everyone to do everything for me and I wasn't sure if I was more angry or upset by that comment. Didn't she know I didn't have a choice? I had no way of doing those things myself. It upset me to think that she saw me as such a burden. Without thinking first, I leaped out of my chair – ignoring the pain – and whacked her over her head with the remote control before trying to run out to my car with my keys. I needed to be away from her.

As she chased after me, I shouted, "I wish you had arthritis just so you could see how it feels and then maybe you wouldn't be so fucking selfish!" "Well, I hope you have it forever and I hope your pains get worse and worse," was the reply and that sent me into a frenzy. I couldn't run, but the adrenaline moved me as fast as I could towards her. As I reached the front door, I went to hit her, having forgotten that my keys were still in my hand and, as my hand approached her face, my key scratched her down the side of her face, just missing her eye. At the time I didn't care; she had hurt me so I hurt her. She deserved it, I thought.

Ilana screamed and cried and called for Mum, who went ballistic and said that I was mad and needed to go back to anger management. She was probably right, but I still didn't think that Ilana's cruel words were justified. The next day, Ilana confronted me and said how upset she was that I had wished arthritis on her. I began to cry and said, "I don't wish it on you, I just wanted you to feel what it's like to be in my shoes for just one day so that you would know how your selfishness upsets me." She too started crying. "You get all the attention all the time so why do you need it from me as well?" she pleaded. "So that's what this is all about, you're jealous. How sick are you? You're jealous of this?" I asked incredulously. "You think I want attention in this way? You're mad. Fine, here, take it." I screamed, whooshing my arms about as if to take the illness out of my body and pass it on to her. "Take my disgusting disease and all the attention that goes with it. I don't want it and if you do then you're crazier than I thought. My little sister looked at me with tears welling up her eyes, "I don't want it and I don't want you to be in pain. I'm sorry." I paused, assessed the situation, then gave her a hug, realising that my words had probably affected her as much as hers had affected me and, more importantly, for the first time I realised that my illness had affected her life just as much as it had mine. I apologised for the things I had said to her and for keying her face and we left it at that.

I was referred back into anger management, this time through my GP. Unfortunately, the session didn't go too well. The therapist pushed all the wrong buttons and sent me into one of my anger-fuelled mood swings. She wasn't like the last therapist I had had: the sweet, understanding lady who hadn't judged and hadn't looked up every line that I uttered in her psychology textbook, as this miserable cow did. I took an instant dislike to her. I hated the generic questions put forward in that stereotypical therapist voice. "So, Lauren, why do you think you get so angry? Where does the rage come from? What do **we** think we can do to solve this rage problem you seem to have?" 'AARRGGHHH! **We** can't do anything', I thought to myself. I wanted to scream. "Err... isn't that obvious? Did you study psychology at all?" I rudely asked as I held back the urge to hit her over the head with one of my crutches. I couldn't be bothered with this. Some girl who had just finished studying psychology at university thought that she could understand me because of what her textbooks said. No, she would never understand, at least not until she had had a bit more life experience. So, I stormed out of my anger management session because my anger management therapist made me angry... what a conundrum.

Things did seem as if they were descending down an everlasting downward slope for a while. I couldn't drive my car anymore, as my left knee was too swollen to push down on the clutch and I didn't have enough money to buy an automatic car. By this point, my car was barely roadworthy anymore. Luminous green fluid leaked out of the exhaust, the passenger door didn't lock and I had to start the car in second gear because first gear didn't work.

I had read in one of the DLA newsletters that people with long-term disabilities might be entitled to a car. I was losing my independence again by not being able to get out and about on my own, even if it was only to drive round to Gemma's or go and buy myself something from the shop.

I had to be receiving higher rate mobility component to get a car, but at the time I was getting the middle rate. I reapplied and someone came round to assess me again. They rejected my application and again awarded me the middle rate. I thought about all the other people out there that probably needed this help more than I did, but then I considered my own position. Aside from those ten short months in which I practically had no signs of arthritis, I had spent a lifetime in pain – without any help from the government, or anybody except my own family. I felt that all I could do now was take this bad situation and use it to my advantage. If I had to live with arthritis from cradle to grave, I bloody well deserved a car that I could actually drive. So I appealed against the rejection.

I was back on crutches most of the time now but because I had such bad pains in my hands, the crutches were hard to use. Finchley Memorial Hospital had provided me with a brand new wheelchair and a bath seat to use at home. The appeal letter came back within six weeks and explained that we would have to appear before a tribunal in Central London. Aba came with me and I asked him to let me do all the talking – he wasn't the best with words. We sat at one side of a table facing about six people. It was intimidating and felt like a board meeting. I decided I would really fight for this car. I genuinely believed that as a twenty-one year-old girl, my independence and sanity depended on this car. I didn't care what car they gave me – I just wanted a way to be able to get myself around without having to rely on my parents. They listened carefully.

I must have said something right because, a few weeks later, I was told that I was being awarded the higher rate mobility component and was now entitled to a car! I was ecstatic. They sent me a list of dealerships that participated in the Motability Scheme in my area and Mum and I went to look at some cars. Neither of my parents had ever had a new car and here I was looking at brand new, shiny cars. A lot of the vehicles I was shown looked like what I would describe to be 'disabled cars', with a raised back to allow a wheelchair to fit and disabled stickers all over them. This was definitely not something I wanted. One thing I always tried to maintain was normality, or at least the perception of it. I may feel different, but the way I looked was important to me. Even as young as five years old, throwing tantrums if one hair was out of place once Mum had put it in a ponytail for school, even then I was trying to maintain normality. It was another characteristic that none of us understood at the time but, as I grew up and Lubina explained my need to always look perfect, we realised that it was a need to hide any evidence of being different. I was working on that, but only on myself and my body. I wasn't ready for a car that gave it all away.

Finally, in the Ford garage in Colindale, I found the car I loved. I wasn't entitled to just any car – it had to be within a certain price range – but there was a black Mazda 3 and it was beautiful. It was bigger than my last car, but not too big, with a boot big enough for my wheelchair and crutches, loads of space inside, and was automatic with power steering. This meant that I wouldn't be in any pain whilst driving. Three days before Christmas 2005, I went to pick up my brand new sparkling car. It was my Christmas present from the government.

I was back seeing Lubina every week and it was lucky that I was getting the small amount of money from DLA because this paid for it, I wouldn't have been able to afford it otherwise. I had forgotten how much she had helped me emotionally and how great I always felt about myself when I came out of her clinic, which had now moved from the Homeopathic Centre into a chiropractic clinic round the corner from my house. It was much more convenient and her treatment room was much brighter and prettier than the dull room in the old place that reminded me so much of my childhood. We worked a lot on the problem I had with my image, and the need to look perfect, and I started seeing a hypnotist, Paul. Paul immediately picked up on my image and relationship issues. My main goal with Paul was to get rid of my vomiting phobia, as it was starting to really affect me. I had even stopped eating certain foods because I was afraid that they might me sick. Paul found where the phobia came from, but seemed to focus more on other emotional issues. He picked up on why I hated my image so much, pretty much in the same way as Lubina had, and he explored where it came from. The more I delved deeper into the past and discovered the reasons behind these issues, the easier they were to deal with. He pointed out that I was not able to be in a relationship because I pushed people away, which was true, but I had never realised it. I pushed them away because I was scared of anyone seeing my imperfections. I was scared of them seeing my swollen joints and finding me vile and couldn't face that sort of rejection. I was terrified of opening up to anyone ever again and telling them about my physical difficulties and emotional insecurities.

I was worried that men would see these and run a mile so, instead of letting that happen, I pushed them away before they got too close. I had been deeply disturbed by what had happened with Michael four years before and, subsequently yet subconsciously, I pushed people away so that that could never happen to me again, but no one knew about that, not even Paul and, at the time, I didn't even realise it myself. Mum always had a go at me every time I met a guy because even if I liked him, I would push him away. Obviously, I denied this and claimed that it was because I didn't like the guy in question. A lesson for anyone who is reading this – mothers know best! I was embarrassed about how I looked and petrified of being rejected because of it. Arthritis isn't exactly the most glamorous of diseases and this made intimacy extremely difficult. There are pamphlets in the arthritis clinics about arthritis and sex, but they don't really help, instead just reassuring you that there are other people going through the same problems. That's great, but it doesn't make you feel sexy. I was so embarrassed by my disease that it stopped me doing things.

After being confined to the house all week, Mum would try to get me out at the weekends. One weekend, Mum suggested some retail therapy to make me feel better and so we went to the Harlequin Centre in Watford to do some shopping. We parked our car at the Mobility car park and, as Mum wheeled me in my chair to the reception area, she saw the electric chairs and scooters and suggested that it might be easier for me to wheel myself around the shops in one of those. I looked at them in disgust; these were contraptions for old people, not for me. Then again, arthritis and wheelchairs were also for old people and I had both of those, so Mum told me that I might as well stop cutting off my nose to spite my face and do myself a favour. So, we took the scooter.

Mum was right. It was easier to press a button and wheel

myself around with ease. I tried to see it as a mini-car. That is until I saw two people I knew and I hid in shame behind Mum. Why was I so embarrassed of something that wasn't my fault?

At the end of my second session with Paul, he told me that my homework that week was to go out without any make-up on for one day. It doesn't seem such a huge task, but I didn't think I would be able to do it. I never left the house without make-up or in casual clothes. I always made an effort to put on nice clothes and make my face look pretty – or as pretty as I thought it could be. But I did it. Realising where my insecurities came from and why I had them gave me a better understanding of myself and people around me. I realised that people really didn't care if I was wearing make-up to go and put petrol in my car, or to physio, and they certainly didn't notice if I was wearing a tracksuit instead of something smarter.

At the same time that Paul was helping me with this, Lubina was helping me to try to open up more to people. I realised that if I met a guy, I would never tell him I had arthritis, as I was too scared. I never told anyone who didn't know me about it. Occasionally, when I was on crutches, the girls would convince me to come to the pub with them and, if someone asked me why I was on crutches, I made up funny stories, saying it was because of playing football, or a dancing injury. These were people from around the area whom I had probably known for years and I realised that they didn't even know I had arthritis, because I had always been too embarrassed to talk about it.

Lubina made me understand that imperfections are what people find endearing and eventually fall in love with. Even top models have imperfections and this is what makes us unique and interesting. She would still ask the question, "What don't you want to see, Lauren?" She believed that my eye would not heal itself until I had seen what it was that I was blocking.

Although I still couldn't 'see' what it was that Lubina was talking about, I began to feel that I was understanding life in a whole new way. Dealing with my emotional issues was helping me all round. Ady always said that everything starts in the mind and I believed that, so I believed that dealing with what was going on, on the inside, would possibly cure what was happening on the outside.

I realised that I didn't need anger management, it had to come from within. I had to let go of my anger, frustration and resentment. These emotions would only lead to more pain and illness. This concept made more sense to me than anything ever had, so I began trying to let it take effect.

I felt as if everything in my life was always stilted, always in limbo. I studied performing arts, but could never go to university. I started doing acting jobs, but couldn't take it further because I couldn't stand up. I studied interior design, but couldn't get a job in the field because I couldn't work let alone use my hands. I was still in a lot of pain, but got myself off the crutches – partly because it hurt my hands too much to use them and also out of sheer determination to walk again and try and make something of my life and be able to finish something, to accomplish something.

I enrolled in an acting course at the London Actors' Workshop in Covent Garden. It was a drama school for actors who already had some experience and it took place every Sunday, and every few weeks we would have a different teacher. It made me think of Rob and I wondered how his acting career was going. Rob, whom I hadn't seen for so many years and yet still felt a connection to. Rob who was the kind, sweet, handsome boy who'd made me feel on top of the world. How different things had turned out and spiraled out of control so soon after our perfect moment a lifetime ago.

The most interesting teacher that taught us at LAW was

Marianna Hill. She had been in The Godfather Part II, one of my favourite films, so I was very excited to meet her. Marianna was eccentric and quirky and wonderful and, for some reason, she took a liking to me. I looked forward to my Sunday acting classes as no one there knew me and it was a way to escape for a few hours. I tried to forget about the pain as much as possible for those three hours and just enjoy being there and I fell in love with acting all over again.

The arthritis manifested itself in many ways to make me aware of the fact that I was not doing something right. One of those ways was Irritable Bowel Syndrome, or IBS. I believed that it was connected to the arthritis because Ady had explained that if I ate white bread and the next day I had pain or swelling in my knee, I wouldn't associate it with the bread, but if I ate white bread and my stomach played up, I would take this into account. My stomach sort of spoke on behalf of my joints, if you like.

My stomach seemed to get very bad really quite quickly. I was either constipated for days on end or I would have the kind of diarrhoea that feels as if it's never going to stop. I was constipated once for fifteen days. I took every type of laxative possible and two suppositories and still nothing. None of it worked, so I went to the doctor and he gave me a special cocktail of laxatives, which caused me to practically live on the toilet for a whole day and night. After that, everything I ate – or even drank – came straight out of me. Gluten and dairy were off limits but everything else was being rejected too. My GP referred me to Dr. Leahy, a gastroenterologist at the BUPA Hospital at Bushey. I finally had private healthcare and this covered anything that wasn't to do with the arthritis, so it was a real luxury being treated in a private hospital. What wasn't such a luxury, though, was what Dr. Leahy had in mind.

Mum and I squeezed each other's hands as we tried not to laugh out loud at how funny all the poo-related words sounded in his heavy Welsh accent. Dr. Leahy told us that because arthritis was an inflammatory disease, he had to check for things like Crohn's and Inflamed Colitis and he could only do this through a colonoscopy.

I wasn't particularly thrilled to have a camera placed where the sun don't shine, but I didn't really have a choice and if I was going to get a private hospital room for once, I couldn't complain.

The night before the procedure, I wasn't allowed to have dinner and had to drink a vile-tasting liquid laxative. This was to wash out the bowel, so that Dr. Leahy could look inside it properly the next day. A friend who had gone through the same procedure had warned me that what happens after you drink this liquid isn't pleasant so I was apprehensive to say the least.

I went to the toilet a couple of times and thought to myself that this wasn't as bad as everyone had made out, having expected to be up all night. I went to bed when I thought it was all over, only to be woken up by the feeling that I was about to shit myself. I ran to the toilet and spent the remainder of the night – and early morning – right there. I got to bed at 6.00am and then had to wake up at 7.00am to go to the hospital.

I arrived feeling tired, hungry and sick and my stomach felt strangely raw. The nurse put Mum and me in my private room and gave me a hospital robe. At least here I don't need to wear a hairnet, I thought to myself. Within an hour I was taken down to surgery, where they sedated me. It wasn't a general anaesthetic and I would know what was going on, but not feel it. Shockingly, however, I did feel it and screamed throughout the whole procedure. I felt something being inserted further and further inside me, wriggling around in my stomach. It was the most bizarre, unnatural feeling that I've ever experienced.

I was brought back to my room and couldn't speak for

hours afterwards. Dr. Leahy came up a few hours later to tell us that thankfully, there was no inflammatory activity in my bowel. The only thing he could put it down to was IBS – which is basically the name they give to any stomach condition when they don't know what's wrong, which, in conventional medicine, is most of the time. He gave me pills that he said would help with the bloating and pain, but the only way I could try to control it was through watching my diet. I was already doing this so wondered what I had put myself through that abhorrent procedure for.

A few weeks later, I landed a part in a play at the Pump House Theatre in Watford. The play, Kindertransport, was about a Jewish woman who had been sent out of Germany as a child during the Second World War on the Kinderstransport trains by her parents, to England. She forgot about her Jewish roots as the years went on and grew up suffering an identity crisis. When her daughter wanted to know more about her life, it all came back to her. I played her daughter.

Rehearsals were held every Tuesday and Friday and it was a part of my life that I looked forward to. It didn't take me long to memorise the script and I was excited to be a part of a play that had so much depth and meaning.

The day before opening night, I awoke to the moment that I had been dreading for years. I had gone completely blind in my right eye. I looked in the mirror and my pupil had turned white where a film was totally covering it. Now, I actually looked blind. A thousand thoughts circulated through my mind before I told Mum and Aba. I had this play to do and it was important. I was also rehearsing for my final showcase at the London Actors' Workshop and couldn't miss that.

I tried to stay as calm as possible and called Mum and Aba into my room. They of course rushed me to Moorfields. Mr. Pavesio said that the cataract had grown numerous layers one over the other and they were covering the eye, which is why I couldn't see and why the eye had gone white. The operation that he had been so reluctant to perform was now essential and urgent as the cataracts were pushing against the optic nerve and the pressure had gone down to zero. It was now the end of February and I urged him to wait until after my play had finished. He agreed and scheduled the operation for the week after my twenty-second birthday – the second week of March.

My music teacher at Performing Arts College, Paul, had always said, 'To be a great stage actor, you need to do two things: remember your lines and not bump into any of the props.' At least I had the first one covered. I would have to deal with the second in another way. I turned up an hour early on the opening night and took myself onto the stage, in the dark. I closed my eyes and walked around the stage and the props, memorising where everything was with my eyes closed. That way, if I couldn't see something on my right-hand side, I would know it was there and wouldn't bump into it. Luckily, I remembered all my lines and didn't bump into any props. At least Paul would say that I was a great stage actress!

The show got off to a great start and I didn't want to get off the stage at the end of each night. On the third night, a group of Kindertransport survivors came to see the play and we enjoyed a question and answer session with them after the show. The fact that they were there, sharing their experiences with us, validated the reason for me trying so hard to be there and finish the run. The hardships that Holocaust survivors had been through were much worse than me losing the sight in one eye. I sat and listened to their stories in awe, thankful for my life.

That weekend, I celebrated my birthday in a Greek restaurant. We ate, danced and threw plates, but I wouldn't let anyone take any pictures, as I didn't want anyone to see my eye and how I looked before the operation. I really believed that the operation was going to work and I wouldn't look like this forever – I couldn't let that happen. Only a few months ago I actually found a picture that someone must have managed to take of me during that week and you can see the eye totally white. I'm kind of glad that that picture was taken so I can see how far I've come.

Zoe and Craig had got engaged and their engagement party was on the Sunday night before my operation, so that was a welcome distraction from the thoughts of what was about to happen on the Tuesday.

I went into Moorfields as an inpatient on the Tuesday morning with my operation scheduled for the Wednesday. I met with a few different doctors, including Mr. Pavesio and one of the top surgeons from the hospital, whose name I can't remember, but I do know that he was a very well-known, well-respected doctor and, if he was the one doing my operation, then it must have been very risky.

I was given my own little room on the ward as I was more prone to infection and I was happy for the privacy. There were some great characters on the ward. Sue bounced out of her room, happy as a clam, and introduced herself straight away. She had had an operation on her eye, but then got an infection and so had to stay in longer and was also given a private room. She laughed as she apologised for not being able to stop farting. There was an elderly French lady in the bed opposite my room, who sat in a chair with her head down on a pillow, tilted to one side. Apparently, she had to stay like this for the fluids in her eye to go in the right direction. I noticed that there were a few women in this position and hoped that I wouldn't have to do that after my operation as it looked extremely uncomfortable.

The other lady I started talking to probably had a more positive attitude than anyone I have ever met. It seems strange that I cannot remember her name, because she made such an impact on me. She introduced herself and said that her operation was on the same day. Soon after, she was given a gown to change into and was told to take off all jewellery as she was going to be taken down to theatre soon. The nurse came to collect her and I will never forget hearing her say, "Hold on nurse, I've just gotta take off my leg." And, she did. She removed her prosthetic leg and carried on as if everything was normal. Everyone on the ward watched in awe at how calm and collected she was and how it all seemed completely normal to her.

When we spoke to her later, she explained that she had very severe diabetes, which caused her to get an infection in her leg. It had turned gangrenous and she was in so much pain that she said she was 'happy for them to take the bloody thing off.' Taking off the foot was not enough and, in the end, she had to have half her leg removed. She told her husband that if he couldn't deal with it, she would understand if he left her but, of course, he didn't and is now her full-time carer. She suffers a huge amount, but takes it all in her stride and is positive about life.

The next day I was nil by mouth and was woken up at 6.00 am by the nurses. Mum and Aba arrived and I had another meeting with the doctors, including my anaesthetist, who just happened to be gorgeous. Unfortunately for me, I was wearing a hospital gown, a hairnet, a pair of 'special' hospital knickers and had a huge black arrow drawn on my face pointing down to my right eye. This was probably not the right time for romance. I told the handsome anaesthetist that I had an awful phobia of being sick, so he had to make sure that they gave me an anti-sickness injection as soon as I came round from the anaesthetic, and they also had to keep me away from any other people in recovery who were being sick. I was very bossy for someone about to have an operation.

I lay on the hospital bed, being wheeled down to theatre

with Mum, Aba and the hot anaesthetist by my side. I was shivering, the way I always did when I was nervous before an operation. For some reason, I always became really cold and shivery before I went into an operating theatre and so I tried to keep my mind positive. The way I saw it – which was the way I had always seen it, but Mr. Pavesio didn't agree – was that the operation would either work or it wouldn't. If I was going to lose the sight anyway – and now I had – what more could I lose by having the operation? But, I was positive. I don't know where it came from but, for some reason, I had always believed that my eye would be OK and I believed it now.

As my parents were worrying more than they'd ever worried, I was calm and collected – aside from the fact that my intense shivering made me look like I was having a seizure. "Good luck," Mum whispered as she was shown out of the room, "we'll be right here when you wake up and we're so proud of you." In my heart of hearts, I genuinely believed that I would be fine. I pictured Ady's face and his calming aura, and imagined what he would say right now to calm me down. As I felt the cold anaesthetic trickle up my arm, Ady's face sent me to a warm, happy place. Mmm, I love the feeling of anaesthetic.

After nearly four hours, I realised that I was waking up in recovery. As I woke up, I started speaking in Hebrew for some odd reason and, in my semi-conscious state, I soon realised that none of the nurses understood me. I tried again. "Anti-sickness injection. Please," I pleaded with the nurse. Within a split second, I felt a deep pang in my thigh and didn't care that it hurt. Even though I didn't feel sick, I was scared that I would be sick at some point and so having the injection would give me one less thing to worry about.

I was brought back up to the ward and, as the anaesthetic started wearing off, I began screaming in pain. The thing about pain is that no matter how much something hurts, it is very rare that you remember what it felt like. It has to be a specific type of pain for you to remember how it actually felt. No matter how much pain I've experienced from arthritis over the years, there have only been three times that a pain has been so awful that I still remember today how it felt. The first was that steroid injection in my knees when I was nine, and this was the second. The third instance happened shortly after this – more of that later.

All I wanted to do was keep my eyes shut but, even with our eyes closed, we tend to blink or move our eyes slightly. If I opened or moved my left eye it would cause the right eye to move slightly and I couldn't control it. Every time my right eye moved, even a tiny bit, I was screaming in pain. It was absolutely excruciating but also frustrating, because I just could not keep my eyes still. We don't realise how much we move our eyes until it is too painful to do so. I was given morphine to relax the muscles in the eye and that helped a bit. This unbearable pain only lasted for the first day, but that was more than enough.

Mum slept next to me on the bed for a while – we were both exhausted – but then my friends turned up. I was really appreciative that they had come to see me, but I was tired and in so much pain that I wasn't in the mood for visitors. They brought flowers and chocolates and didn't stay too long because they could see how much pain I was in.

When I was advised that I should eat something, I only fancied sweet food. Because of the IBS, I had cut out gluten, dairy and sugar and had not touched either for about six months. However, all I wanted now were those little caramel waffles from Starbucks and then, the next day, bagels. A little bit of what you fancy does you good, Mum always says. Luckily, my stomach behaved itself for a while – maybe it was giving me a break to recover. Mum was of the opinion that the colonoscopy had washed out the problems that had been causing the cramps and diarrhoea and my stomach was clean again, which is why it was accepting foods that it had rejected before. None of these theories were right, but again, I explain it all at the end.

Before I had the operation, the pressure in my eye had dropped to 0. This is extremely dangerous as the correct pressure is about 12. We hoped that if the operation worked, the pressure would go back up. The elderly French lady had a dangerously high pressure, so we joked that she would give me some of hers and that way we would balance each other out.

Ilana arrived to see me and left with Mum and Aba at about 8:30. The patch and bandages would be coming off my eye the next day and so I needed to sleep.

The next day, the doctors came round to the ward very early and, although I had wanted Mum and Aba to be there when the patch came off, the doctors began their rounds at 7:45. Assisted by the nurses, Mr. Pavesio removed the patch. My eye was still closed and I was too nervous to open it. The nurses started to clean the eye and, as I slowly opened it, I saw a cotton bud heading towards me. I fell to the floor and passed out. Although it was still very blurry, I could see an object for the first time since I was seventeen and I think it was hard for my brain to accept, which is why I felt so strange. I came around and the nurses put me back into my bed, opened the windows to give me some air and raised my legs on top of lots of pillows and I lay there for a while, trying to compose myself. At this moment Mum and Aba walked in and I sobbed uncontrollably, shouting, "I can see!" over and over again.

No one knew what to make of this, as the doctor hadn't had a chance to check me yet and my parents were in shock. Mr. Pavesio explained that in normal cataract operations, they remove the lens and replace it with a fake one. In my case, the eye had been too inflamed to put anything else in there so, when they removed all the layers of the cataract, they also removed the lens and inserted a type of gas into my eye, but they had not replaced the lens. He explained that, if I did have vision, it would be as a camera would be without a lens, unfocused and blurry. He also said that the operation had been a success. Many of his colleagues had thought that it would fail but, somehow, against all odds, I came through it just fine and my pressure had even gone up to two. Mum and Aba were over the moon. Because the doctors themselves had been so worried about carrying out the operation, my parents too had been very apprehensive.

I lay on the bed, assessing the world around me with my new 'vision'. I kept remembering seeing the cotton bud heading for my eye and thinking 'I can see that'. Mr. Pavesio had said that in order for this operation to work, I would have to take oral steroids to keep the inflammation down and I had no choice in the matter this time. I hadn't argued, because I had desperately wanted him to do the operation and so I had reluctantly agreed to take the steroids for two weeks before and two weeks after the operation.

Because I had already been taking the steroids for two weeks, I was starting to feel the effects. The palpitations, the sweats and the increase in arthritis symptoms were all present. I decided to keep quiet because I only had to take them for another two weeks and then it would all be over, but my joints definitely felt strange in the same way that they had the last time. It was a different sort of pain and I was itchy all the time, constantly scratching my skin. I could feel the chemicals swimming around my blood like my blood was itchy. Heroin addicts have the same symptom. Chemicals were chemicals in my eyes and it didn't matter if I was taking steroids or heroin, I wasn't happy at all about it.

I was discharged on the Friday afternoon after being seen by Mr. Pavesio, plus a few other doctors and some medical students who, for some reason, found my case fascinating. Mr. Pavesio seemed concerned to justify the reason for not having carried out the operation before when, as it turned out, if he had, it would have been successful. I assured him that it wasn't his fault and that he was just being cautious but, up to this day, he still tries to justify his actions. He was just doing his job and a doctor's job is not always about using their intuition. I believe what happened to my eye to be one of the miracles that have happened to me over the years. The doctors had decided not to perform the operation and so nature intervened and made the eye so bad that the operation was forced upon us. This is why I believe that everything happens for a reason. I also know that part of the reason why this operation – the one that the doctors were so afraid to do – succeeded is because of my genuine belief that it would.

The day that Mum and Aba took me home from hospital, everything seemed different. I had to rest, but I felt as if this operation had awoken all my senses. It was only March and so not too warm, but I wanted the windows open so that I could feel and smell the air. The colours in my room appeared vibrant and beautiful. The grass looked the most stunning shade of green and the sky a striking blue. Even food tasted different. I don't know if it was the fact that I could see out of my eye that made so much difference to my senses, but everything around me felt wonderful.

A few days after I came home, it rained heavily. For some reason, I wanted to go and stand in the rain. Mum said that if that's what I felt like doing, I should do it. I walked outside in my pyjamas and slippers and just stood, letting the rain soak me. Mum and I were both laughing and crying uncontrollably, as if hundreds of emotions that had been lost inside us for so many years were being released. I don't know why I had the urge to do this, but I certainly felt a different person from the young girl who had sat in the rain, on her own, one cold and miserable night four and a half years earlier.

Easter came and we celebrated Passover. We had been invited round to family friends for dinner for the first night of Passover. I started feeling a bit strange during dinner so I went in another room to lie down. We left at about 11.00pm and I went to sleep, only to awake at 4:30 in the morning facing the single most painful experience of my life. Both knees were in agonizing pain. Throughout my years, although I've done my fair share of moaning, I've managed to keep relatively quiet while in pain, but this particular morning I screamed until I could scream no more. It felt as if someone was sanding the bones in my knees with a chainsaw and however much an exaggeration that may sound, I can assure you that 'excruciating' was an understatement. I genuinely believed that I was dying, or would die from the pain alone.

My parents sat with me trying to calm me down, but I couldn't. I just needed the pain to stop. They gave me painkillers that I'd been given from the hospital, but they weren't enough. I was wriggling and writhing and couldn't stop screaming. Even Ilana, who usually slept through absolutely anything, woke up and came in to try and help.

Aba went downstairs and I heard him praying. He was praying in a way that I had never heard him do outside of Synagogue. As he prayed, he cried and I heard him pleading with God to make my pain go away. I was in too much pain to concentrate but it was emotional and made my own emotional state even more volatile. Mum and I sat on my bed crying, as she held my hand while I screamed and wriggled to the sound of Aba praying.

After about an hour of screaming, Mum called an ambulance and sat with me on the way to hospital while Aba followed in the car. Ilana didn't come, but instead went back to bed, which set off an alarming realisation in my mind later on; me being in pain was completely customary to her. I had noticed this before. I knew that if my friends' siblings were ill, they would be around them doing everything they could to help but Ilana wasn't even fazed. I used to get annoyed with my sister for not helping me when I was in pain but that day I started realising that this was because she knew no different. Throughout her whole life she had seen me in pain, so she didn't know what it was like to have a sister who wasn't sick and had got used to blocking it out. That's why on that day, when she went back to bed, I stopped being angry with her.

The paramedics gave me gas and air, which was great for the few seconds it lasted. As I put the mask over my mouth, the pains faded and I couldn't stop laughing but as soon as I took it off, the laughter turned into screams as the pain returned.

At the hospital, they could come up with no explanation whatsoever as to the cause of the pain. It was clearly not normal arthritis pain. One thing and one thing only came to my mind – it was the steroids. I was now too drowsy from the cocktail of pills they had given me to think too deeply about it, but Mum and I both knew the reason. I was just thankful that it had finally passed. This was the third instance of acute pain that I mentioned earlier and was, by far, the worst.

It took me a few weeks to recover from the knee pain as it exhausted me so much – I literally slept for days after that.

Jojo mentioned to Mum that she had heard of a special spiritualist doctor who was supposed to have helped people with all kinds of diseases. He was due to give a talk at a church in Borehamwood and so a few weeks after my knee incident, we decided to go along. As usual, we were up for trying anything and spiritualism was not something I was unfamiliar with, although we'd never been part of a church congregation.

We got there early and sat in the front seats. There were posters and testimonials everywhere about how this doctor/priest/healer had healed people and I began to feel intrigued. "This isn't going to be one of those gospel Church 'hallelujah, she's healed!' type of things, is it?" I asked Mum anxiously. "I really don't know, sweetheart," she replied, and at that moment a woman came on stage and started to talk.

I know that I wasn't exactly 'Miss Sociable' at that moment but, as the congregation started singing hymns, I thought to myself that there were other things I could be doing on a Saturday night – even if it was only staying at home to watch The X Factor. All those people sitting around us seemed to be regulars as they knew every song by heart and every so often, people around the Church would throw their arms in the air and shout 'Praise the Lord!' I felt like an extra in Forrest Gump. Mum and I began to giggle and Jojo, being the polite lady that she is, told us to be quiet. We did try, honestly we did, but it was too much like something out of a movie.

The hymns finished and the doctor/priest/healer was introduced. The very average-looking middle-aged man began speaking in a loud, deep voice that touched the back of the room effortlessly. "Who… needs to be healed?" he asked, very slowly. "Who… needs to feel the power of the Lord's hand?" OK, now I was scared. This really was like a scene from a movie and any minute someone would go up on stage, he would put his hand on them and that person would claim to be healed.

Oh shit, he was looking at me. He noticed my crutches. Shit, shit, shit. "Young lady, you look like you need to experience healing at the hands of the Lord. Come up here and join us! Agnes, help the young lady onto the stage." As Agnes, an overweight and rather malodorous lady who was far too excited, helped me onto the stage, the whole audience clapped and cheered and I looked back at Mum and Jojo, hoping that they would rescue me. They didn't. I was now on stage with this weird guy, fat Agnes and another highly unfortunate looking lady. "What disease plagues your body, child?" he asked, with his eyes closed. "Arthritis," I whispered. "ARTHRITIS," he shouted, loud enough to make me jump, "at such a young age," he tutted, and shook his head. "The Lord Jesus Christ can heal you, my child," and, with that, he put his hand on my head and shook it fiercely. My crutches were starting to wobble. Again, he shocked me with a loud outburst, "Do you believe in the Lord, the only Son of God, Jesus Christ? Say 'I believe in Jesus Christ' and he will surely heal you, child." "HALLELUJA!" shouted a voice from the audience, followed by, "Boy, have they got the wrong girl" from the vicinity of where my mum was sitting. I looked around at the faces of all these firm believers, waiting at the edge of their seats for a miracle, and I couldn't think of anything to say except, "...but I'm Jewish." I heard Mum chuckle and Jojo put a hand over her mouth in disbelief. The doctor/ priest/healer replied, "Christ will still heal you, child." Well, Christ was a Jew, after all. "Lord, take the Devil out of this young person, LORD!" He was now shouting at the top of his voice while still vigorously shaking my head, now with both hands. "Release the evil of the Devil from her body, take the Devil out of this child now, Lord."

'Praise the Lords' and 'Hallelujahs' were flying round the room like bats awoken from their slumber in a Romanian cave and I felt like a prize idiot – albeit a bit emotional. He asked Agnes to take my crutches away as he held both my hands and said, "Child, can you walk?" 'Well, of course I can walk; you are holding my hands, you idiot' – is what I wanted to say. But I nodded and Agnes and the unfortunate looking lady took an arm each and helped me to walk slowly across the stage. He started shouting "Praise the Lord, the Lord has healed," and everyone clapped, shouted and sang. The idiots. The two women supporting me were no different from my crutches, so what was the difference now? There was none. My legs still hurt and Jesus had not healed me. I let them have their moment and then asked for my crutches back. Agnes reluctantly gave them back to me and I walked as fast as I could to the toilet, where I called Charlie in fits of laughter. Mum and Jojo met waited for me outside the toilet and we sneaked out of the hall, followed by people asking about my 'miracle' and quickly got away.

The following week there was an article in the local newspaper about a healer in Borehamwood who had healed a young girl with arthritis and she now no longer needed her crutches. We had a good laugh out of it, though. After all, if you can't laugh at yourself, life would be pretty boring.

The experience at the Church didn't make me believe any less in my ability to get better. I just saw it as an extremely amusing experience that would be entertaining to talk about in years to come.

Chapter 11

Finding GRACE

A few months after the operation, and once the eye had started to recover, I was referred to the Contact Lens Clinic at Moorfields. They tested the vision in my eye and gave me a lens. Because I no longer had a real lens in my eye, my vision was as Mr. Pavesio said it would be – blurry and unfocused. The contact lens they gave me was supposed to make the vision a lot clearer. After two custom-made lenses, the third one worked. It was amazing to put the lens in and be able to see, but there was a slight problem. My brain had gotten so used to not being able to see out of that eye that I became dizzy and disorientated every time I wore the lens. They told me it was a refraction problem and it was normal but that I'd have to persevere with it until my brain adjusted. Every day I'd put it in and get all dizzy and disorientated and it would make me feel sick. I couldn't drive with it in and I didn't want to be out too long if I had it in so it was kind of hard to adjust to 'normal' life with it. After a few months my brain still was not adjusting to it and I eventually gave up. I didn't really care too much anyway. The operation had worked and I hadn't lost my eye. I can deal with only seeing out of one eye, as long as the other one is still there.

It took a while for the steroids to get out of my system and

I didn't feel that great for a good few months. My final showcase at the London Actors Workshop was taking place in April. Although I was back on crutches most of the time, as the incident with my knees had left them weak and unstable, I decided that the actress in me would have to take over for the night of the showcase.

The piece that had been chosen for me was a comedy duologue with another student, Kevin. The showcase was taking place in a theatre in Kings Cross and the whole class spent all day rehearsing. I was on my crutches all day and, as 7.30 pm approached, I was getting extremely tired. I tried to buck up and forget about it while I did my hair and make-up.

Kevin and I waited backstage for our turn and just before they called us out I decided to lay my crutches down and just pretend I wasn't in pain. I spent the remainder of my short time on stage blocking out the pain and walking as if nothing was wrong.

Our duologue was a comedy piece and we got a standing ovation and made everyone laugh. That feeling of making people laugh (or cry or whatever it is you're trying to achieve) was amazing. I never wanted to get off the stage, I just wanted to keep doing whatever it was that made people recognise a talent in me. I wanted recognition and any actor or performer will tell you that. We want to know every last bit that you enjoyed, what you enjoyed about it, what exact feelings it made you feel. It isn't enough to just say, 'you were really good.' Performers have big egos and need acceptance constantly and the laughter that night was acceptance for me.

The other piece of recognition I achieved from that performance was particularly interesting. After the show, I was told that there were some agents in the audience and one of them wanted to speak to me. His name was Roger De Courcey – the same Roger De Courcey who was the famous ventriloquist from the '70s. He was now an agent and I went to meet him a few days later and he took me on. I had some more headshots done, joined up to Spotlight again and felt like things might be happening for once.

I started feeling better in myself, again, so I decided to start working. I wanted to get a part-time job so that I could still audition and spend time on getting better, and I knew jumping straight back into full-time work wouldn't allow for that but I also knew I had to get back into 'normal' life to aid my recovery.

I got a job at the crèche in the LA Fitness gym in Finchley. I had to undergo police checks and first aid training and the rest of the training was done on the job by Pam, our manager.

Working in the crèche was perfect for me at that time. I found working with babies to be therapeutic and good for the soul and I had plenty of free time left over also.

During this time, I worked on myself and my body and tried to figure out ways to make myself healthy again. I had already learnt how powerful the mind could be, so all I had to do was put this into practice. I was meditating daily, doing lots of visualisation and positive thinking exercises and started reading books by Louise Hay, Deepak Chopra and Dr. Brian Weiss. The Louise Hay books helped me a lot, as her main theory was the basis of what I was trying to do – believe that everything starts in the mind and therefore believe that your mind can mend things. Deepak Chopra also follows the same beliefs and the Weiss books gave me more insight into spirituality and helped me believe that everything happens for a reason. His books examine regression into past lives – something I have always been interested in – and he talks about soul mates and soul families. My view on organised religion has been drastically altered over the years and my beliefs are a pretty different to those of most people I know, but what I do know is that it is important to believe in *something*, to know that there is a god – despite how you may want to label of perceive that – a powerful entity beyond what our five senses can allow us to acknowledge. If you believe in nothing, how can you ever believe in the power of healing? What do skeptics think the reason is that some people with the same illness die, and some recover, when they are on the same medication? Science can only go so far.

I would say that at this stage, I was still at the very beginning of my learning; I was starting to open up to new ideas and concepts, to acknowledge that there was much more to healing and the body than meets the eye and although the next decade was about to teach me so much more, that journey was beginning and I became much more involved and interested in other forms of spirituality. I visited the Buddhist Centre in Holloway Road to take part in group meditations. This showed me that the force behind a collective positive energy being sent out to the universe could be astounding. I took more of an interest in nature and how we are connected to nature and with all the meditating and tree hugging I became known as somewhat of a hippy. I wasn't bothered by titles; all I knew is that I wasn't angry anymore.

We found other supplements along the way and tried them all – still not finding the right balance but being willing to try it all to eventually learn the right way – from apple cider vinegar (which I still swear by) and molasses, to olive leaf extract and Korean Red Ginseng.

The IBS started improving after I'd been taking a very good brand of probiotics for about a month and the less frequent trips to the toilet made life much more comfortable.

In time, I ditched the crutches totally and life seemed like it was going in the right direction. By my second year at LA Fitness, I'd work in the crèche in the morning, then do a few hours of membership sales in the sales office for some extra cash after lunch. Some of the staff at the gym were offered the chance to take a fitness instructor course and I decided to take it. It wasn't a career choice but it would certainly do me no harm to learn more about the body.

I remembered how overdoing it not so long ago had not helped in the slightest so I only worked four days and Fridays were dedicated to physio and hydro. Andre had left rheumatology to join the main outpatient's physio so I was assigned to Christina, the head of rheumatology physio. Christina found me quite hard to understand and although she was a good physio, and we had a lot in common personally, we also clashed a lot. She had no belief whatsoever in natural therapies. She believed that drugs were the way forward and deviating from that would only cause long-term problems. I was, of course, on the complete other side of the fence. She kept advising me to take the drugs that Dr. Keat was offering and I didn't understand why anyone would advise this to someone who was clearly getting better, not worse.

What I found even more frustrating than Christina – she was medically trained after all and her views were as they were because they had been taught to her like that – were the other arthritis sufferers with whom I took hydro classes. I looked around the pool and noticed just how different I was. I had always worried about looking different to 'normal' people, but what I never realised was how exponentially different I was to other arthritis sufferers. *I* was the odd one out in this crowd. It turned out, I looked normal after all. I was one of the only ones there who didn't have any deformities, the only one without a puffy face from steroids and one of few who didn't have osteoporosis from taking steroids for so many years. I'd had a bone density scan a few weeks previously and my results shocked Dr. Keat. The scan showed my bone density to be the same as that of a healthy twenty-two year old when most people in my situation had severe joint damage by now. *Unusually healthy*, was how they referred to my joints. I was also one of the only people in the pool who had not had a joint replacement. These were not good odds. I started to realise how lucky I was. But was it luck or was it the fact that I was the only one who was treated with complementary therapies? The numbers spoke for themselves.

I knew that it was down to not spending a lifetime on immunosuppressants, steroids and disease modifying drugs, and instead using homeopathy and other alternative therapies to aid the body into recovery. It may not have cured me (at this point, anyway), but it had sure made me healthier than everyone else in my situation. Surely that wasn't a coincidence? (I don't believe in coincidences anyway.)

I tried to speak to some of the girls about it; we'd grown up together after all, we could be open with each other. Apparently not. I was totally shocked by their reactions. They were not interested. They had such negative attitudes towards anything 'alternative' that they weren't even willing to give it a go. I was standing there, sans crutches, in my swimming costume, looking fairly normal, walking in and out of the hydro pool as I pleased, while most of the others were hoisted in and out.

They were all too 'scared' to try something different and didn't want it to 'interfere' with their medications, which I'd happily understand if their medications were working but they were all so ill! It made no sense to me! What was there to interfere with?? They'd been on medication after medication since childhood and the arthritis only got worse and was followed by other illnesses brought on by the meds. Why couldn't they see that? Their attitudes angered and frustrated me. They were all so ill, but were not willing to change their thought patterns or try something new and I just couldn't understand why. I began to realise that what Ady said was right. Some people use their illness as a crutch. They are so used to having this illness that it becomes who they are and gives them a purpose so they have no desire to get better. Some of them even enjoyed the fact that they had an excuse not to work and not one of those girls had ever even though it possible to make something of themselves and there was no one there pushing them forward, encouraging them to be more than they'd allowed themselves to be until this point. This would be their lives forever and they had succumbed to that but not me. I decided to stop going to hydro after that and went swimming instead.

I decided to look on the Internet for websites about young people with arthritis. Daily use of the internet was still fairly new so I had never thought to look it up before but then I came across GRACE – which stands for Give Rheumatoid Arthritis Children Encouragement – a website that was run by a family in Blackpool whose daughter, Bekie, was diagnosed with arthritis when she was fifteen months old. The family wanted to raise money to build a hydro pool in their local hospital and that is what encouraged them to start the charity.

I left a message on the guestbook and within a few hours, Bekie replied. She was now thirteen years old and suffered terribly. Bekie and I exchanged emails about our stories and she asked if she could call me. I had a lovely conversation with her and her mother. They had stopped fundraising for the moment as they didn't have time. I suggested that maybe, if I helped out, it would take some of the pressure off them and they were delighted.

I wanted to raise money for children with arthritis but I didn't want the money to go into pharmaceutical research or chemical medications. I wanted to raise awareness into the fact that it happened to children and young people, not just the elderly. I also wanted to raise money for research into uveitis, in the hope that situations like mine could be prevented in the future. The other thing I wanted to do was raise the profile of alternative therapies and, maybe, if it was possible, look into opening an IPEC clinic in the UK. I had big ideas, for which the Boyd family was not yet ready, but they invited us to Blackpool to meet them. We agreed, because as well as feeling comfortable talking to people with whom we had so much in common, it would be great for Mum to be able to talk to another mother in the same situation.

We stayed with them for the weekend and they were a lovely family. We got on with them really well and had a great time, but it hurt me to see Bekie the way she was. The steroids had had such a bad effect on her growth that she was tiny – I couldn't believe she was thirteen years old as she could have passed for eight. Her face was puffy from the steroids and she didn't like what the disease had done to her hands and feet. Bekie's little body had been destroyed by the years of strong medication and all I wanted to do was to tell her that there were other options. They listened to my story and my views on alternative medicine and diet and took in what we said, but were reluctant to try this route, just like the girls in hydro. It took Bekie near on eight years until she told me she wished she had have listened to me then, when she was thirteen. At twenty-one, she has just realised that the medications never helped and she is still the same as she has always been and she is now going down the holistic route with my help and perhaps if she would have started at thirteen instead of twenty-one, she might have been able to enjoy her teenage years more.

I think much of the reason for people's reluctance was the fear of what would happen if they came off their medication. If they were this unhealthy while they were on it, it was hard to imagine what would happen when they stopped. Firstly, I said, alternative treatments can be used alongside anything else you are taking and, secondly, it was the medication that actually made me worse. What if this was the case for Bekie too? I didn't want to sound as if I was preaching and so didn't discuss it too much, instead trying to make them see that there were other options if they wanted to explore them. I wanted to use the charity to make other people aware of this.

We kept in touch after we returned home. I began to look into ways to raise awareness and, just at that time, received a call from someone from the National Rheumatoid Arthritis Society (NRAS), who had been given my number by Tania.

There was a Parliamentary event being held at the House of Commons for young people with arthritis and they asked if I would like to talk. I was ecstatic. I had no problem speaking in front of people and, if it was going to help raise awareness of JRA, then I was more than game. Bekie's family were hoping to come too but in the end the practicalities of travelling down from Blackpool meant that unfortunately they couldn't make it.

I bought a new, fairly conservative outfit for the occasion; a grey pinafore dress with a black polo-neck underneath and black tights. As Aba drove us into the Houses of Parliament, I was really excited. I'd never done anything like this before and it felt really important.

We were taken on a tour around the Houses of Parliament and through Westminster Hall which is over a thousand years old. After that, we went to the House of Commons room in which our event was taking place. Before the event actually started, we met a lot of very interesting people, including some who work for ARC (Arthritis Research Campaign) and NRAS (National Rheumatoid Arthritis Society), all of whom seemed uninterested in my story and were reluctant to hear any more about my 'strange, alternative lifestyle'.

The MP hosting the event was David Amess. He was backing the cause for awareness into childhood arthritis and was very interested in everything I had to say.

On a table were a number of books, leaflets and pamphlets about children with arthritis. We were given a book by ARC and Mum got really emotional. It was a book for parents and families of children with arthritis and aimed to help from the minute of diagnosis right through to adulthood. There were so many things in that book that would have helped my parents twenty years ago and it upset Mum to know that something so simple could have helped so much. It wasn't so much the technical information but more about its explanation of how the illness would affect siblings – which was clearly the case with Ilana – and how it causes irrational mood swings, the need to be perfect and how some teenagers who have been through a childhood with arthritis will rebel. If only this book had been available all those years ago, everything would have made a lot more sense and things could have possibly been prevented.

The Jewish Chronicle came along wanting to write an article about me and asked about my experiences. I told them about Ady and IPEC and how I have tried to do my best to help myself.

Quite a few people spoke but, during one speech, Mum whispered to me to look around the room at all the other sufferers. It was the same as at the hydro pool. There must have been about forty arthritis sufferers under the age of thirty and, yet again, I was the odd one out, the only one who didn't look 'arthritic' and this really started to hit home now. My difference was more widespread than just alongside the ten arthritis sufferers in the hydro pool; I was different from nearly every arthritis sufferer I had ever met. No matter what the doctors, physiotherapists or anyone else said when claiming that it might be a coincidence, I now knew the truth and nothing would ever change that.

I came away from the House of Commons that day feeling proud of myself for how much I'd achieved and how far I'd come, and thankful to my parents for believing that the alternative therapies would work at a time when few others believed in them. But I felt sad for all the other young people going through what I had been through, but with no way out and no belief that it would ever get better.

I called Bekie and told her about the day's events but I realised that a charity raising awareness into JRA wasn't what I wanted to do. I didn't want to do what all the other arthritis charities were doing. At the Parliamentary event, reps from the big arthritis charities spoke and all their talks revolved around the drugs and which ones to take. I didn't believe that this was the best route to follow when advising people, but at the time I wasn't aware that these charities were backed by the pharmaceutical companies they were recommending. Healthcare did not escape capitalism, despite what some people might think. I knew I had to find my own way when it came to raising awareness but I wasn't there yet.

The article in the Jewish Chronicle created a buzz around my area and I started receiving phone calls, not only from people we knew who wanted to congratulate me, but also from other arthritis sufferers who were getting in touch with me for advice. The author of the article called me nearly every day to ask if she could give my number out. I became a sort of agony aunt for arthritis sufferers and was happy to help and to be someone who these people felt they could turn to. After all, I, more than anyone, knew what it felt like to need to speak to someone who really understands.

Two years after starting work at LA Fitness, I was still there. My condition was up and down and unlike most other cases of arthritis. If I got a flare, I would work on it using all my weird and wonderful methods and usually it would go down. Sometimes it took longer than others, but I did OK. The only problem with looking healthy was that a lot of people at work didn't understand what I actually went through. I admit that I probably didn't talk to them about it enough, but I didn't want to bore people. When I came in on crutches for a week, they understood that it might take me longer to do things but if the next day I came in without them, it was as if all of a sudden I didn't have arthritis and was able to do everything, just because they could see the crutches and without them I had an invisible illness.

I guess I sound as if I am contradicting myself, because I never wanted to look or seem different but, at the same time, I suppose I needed an understanding with the people I worked with as I was with them a lot of the time. No matter how understanding my friends were, this was always the case with them too. If I seemed OK, then no one realised that I was probably still in pain. These things got frustrating but, if I wanted to live a normal life, I just had to deal with it and be happy that my condition was so much better than that of so many others.

The good thing about LA Fitness was that my job was so flexible. I basically did my own hours, had Fridays off for physio and didn't have to work at the weekends. The fear of working in a place without that flexibility if I had a flare was what kept me at LA Fitness for over two and a half years. But I knew I had to bite the bullet at some point and leave to go and do the things I'd always wanted to do. Roger hadn't managed to get me that many auditions and although I tried things to help along the way, it wasn't an option to stop working completely. The better I got, the more pressure I was under to earn money and contribute. It was a tough decision, especially since being an actress had been my dream since I was fourteen, but life got in the way one too many times and I had to trust that that was for a reason and it wasn't meant to be, so decided it was time to say goodbye to that dream and take my life out of the constant limbo it always seemed to be in. As long as I was doing something creative I knew I'd be happy and the only things I'd ever studied or tried to work in were creative jobs. Acting was a dream, and I'll always have that dream, but it was time to start my adult life in a career and that career would be interior design. If I were to get experience in this field, then I couldn't really leave it any longer – I was already twenty-three.

I joined a design recruitment agency and, within a week, Oliver from the agency called to tell me that I had an interview at a company in Old Street. I was both excited and nervous about the interview, as I really didn't know what to expect, but I went along in a lovely new outfit and took with me my portfolios from college. As I walked in, I instantly felt that it was a place where I would love to work. It was a big open-plan studio, with huge windows and lots of light. All the fabric swatches hung in one corner and there was a shelf full of interior design books. The company was called Callender Howorth, and was run by Mark Howorth who had opened the company about ten years before, and his creative director, Drew. Three others worked there and, as I sat being interviewed by Mark, I became less nervous. I left feeling invigorated and, within two hours, Oliver called to tell me that they had offered me the job.

A few days before, I had gone into a brand new furniture shop that imported furniture from the Far East and also offered a design service. They also offered me a job. I wasn't sure which one to take, as they were both offering the same salary but, in the end, I decided that the studio in Old Street was much more my style and I knew it would give me the experience I needed.

I couldn't have been more right. It was a fantastic company to work for. I worked mostly with Drew and he and Mark were both great fun to be around. There was so much to learn, but it made me realise that when it comes to designing you either have an eye for it or you don't. I learned about the different types of styles, the best places to buy furniture and fabrics and also the boring but very important things, such as budgeting and schedules.

Mark and Drew had opened a sister company in Nice, in the South of France where they designed homes for people from England who bought holiday homes out there. I was lucky enough to be able to travel there a few times with them. It was a beautiful place and we had a really good time. One time Mark took all of us from the office for the weekend, un-work related and threw a party at his house and we went to a club afterwards. I also came to see how the design differed out there. People who had homes in London usually kept them quite traditional, in neutral colours and with furniture that wasn't that over the top but, in France, they were willing to experiment and have a bit more fun with their holiday homes and this made it a lot more interesting for us.

I was able to experiment with different colours, styles, fabrics, textures and furniture and discovered my love for one-off pieces, re-inventing furniture by re-upholstering, and eclectic styles that still looked elegant and homely.

Zoe's wedding soon came along and we travelled with to Prague for her hen weekend and then celebrated their wedding at the Dorchester Hotel in Park Lane. It was a fabulous evening.

At work, we were concentrating on a major project in Switzerland. An extremely wealthy businessman had hired the well-known architect, Richard Rogers, to design his state-of-the-art ski chalet, and Callender Howorth were taken on to design the interiors. I travelled there every few weeks with Mark and Drew to administer the finishing touches. We furnished the four-storey chalet from top to bottom and also took care of the final styling, including accessories. We were on the go from morning until night and the hectic schedule and all the travelling really took it out of me but I carried on. I was travelling around Europe, designing villas in Nice and ski chalets in Switzerland – it was a dream. But arthritis found a way of destroying all my dreams and I started to get pains again in my knees and hands. I hoped that it was just a blip, but day-to-day tasks began to become very difficult and, as the days went on, it seemed to be getting worse. I was finding it really hard to grip anything and would make huge mistakes in the studio when I was asked to cut anything with scissors. Every day, it got harder and harder to hold a pen and I began to be extremely thankful for computers.

It didn't take long for the flare-up to take full effect and within a few weeks things were really difficult. My right shoulder was playing up and, yet again, the simple daily task of getting out of bed in the morning was getting too hard to cope with. I went to Dr. Keat who said that, although he couldn't do anything about my swollen fingers unless I wanted to take one of the dreaded medications, my left knee and right shoulder had so much fluid in them that they would have to be drained and have steroid injected into them. It still amazes me how flare-ups can take effect so rapidly. One week I was jetting off all over Europe and the next I had enough fluid in my joints to fill up a water bottle.

I spoke to Mark about it and he seemed quite understanding, but I knew it would be a problem. The plan was to take a week off to have the injections and recover from them but that one week turned into three as I was just too ill to go back to work. At the end of the third week, I received a letter from Mark telling me they had decided that it was not going to work anymore.

I am sure that during the last few weeks that I was with them, I wasn't able to do my job properly, and a company like that needed someone who was able to take on all the extra work. I was upset that I had lost my job, but I understood that they needed someone who was there all the time.

I felt like I was back to square one and I just felt very down. I just couldn't understand how this was happening to me again. I knew as well as anyone that there was no point in asking 'why me?', as this wouldn't bring me any answers.

So how, I wondered, could I turn this latest situation into a positive? I tried to stay as calm and collected as possible, continued with my meditations and concentrated on being healthy, then the idea just came to me. I'd always thought about having my own business so that was the answer. If I ever wanted to be independent it really was the only option. Although I was positive and didn't like to think of the arthritis as something that defined me, it was always going to be there and I would get flare ups every so often so what was I going to do – leave a job every time I had a flare up? No way!

So LV Interiors was born. I put hours of hard work into opening my own business. I had to find an accountant and go through all the logistics of actually opening a business, but more important than that, I had to go through the process of setting up an interior design company and this is no easy task. I took as much knowledge as I could from the experience I gained at Callender Howorth and just got on with it.

I did a one year stint as a radio presenter while I was building up the business, always finding ways for performing to integrate itself back into my life somehow.

I had realised that really, having my own business was always my only option, it had just taken me until now to realise what had to be done. It would mean that no matter what happened and how many flare ups I had, I would be my own boss, no one could fire me and I'd never have to feel bad. If I could work from home, this was half of the pressure taken off me as part of the problem during a flare up was getting into town for 8.30am. I knew I had enough motivation to get up early – even if I was working from home – and work hard to make this happen. This along with the right attitude and obviously the ability to design houses, would give me what I'd always been looking for – success and fulfilment.

By a stroke of luck, my first project presented itself the following month.

Epilogue

Just the Beginning

That flare-up soon subsided but then I had one that was unlike the others. With all the others they came, stayed for about a month, then went, and I put that down to the power of homeopathy, working its magic while the flare-up was present, helping my body through the worst. I assumed that was the best I would get; one or two flares a year that lasted for a month or so. I didn't dare to think about the arthritis ever fully going away, I knew no different. But then I got a flare that lasted for three years. It was the longest flare I'd ever had and no matter what I did, it just didn't go away but all the lessons I'd learned up until then were just scratching the surface. I had so much to learn about health and how to be healthy long-term, how to get rid of an illness instead of treating symptoms and this is now part of my life's work.

I ran my interior design business successfully for seven years until my work as a campaigner and writer left no time for it and I made the decision to prioritise what I thought was important. It is always something I can revisit in the future, but for now, I have been fortunate enough to find other passions and interests that not only keep me busy, stimulated and excited about life, but that help people also.

So what did I learn and what do I now try to teach others?

Well, here goes: I had to get as ill as I got for as long as I did – those last three years – to really work to find the answers, to dig beneath the surface and look for other ways, ways that would not deal with flare-ups when they came, but ways that would lead me to cure myself fully and prevent other illnesses and it took a long time, but with a little bit of luck, a lot of hard work, and a fair amount of perseverance, I eventually found those answers.

My first lesson was this: the medical establishment in the western world is not set up to cure disease, it is a business; a huge, multi-billion dollar business and the most important lesson I ever learned was that if we were all healthy, these businesses would fail and nothing and no one will allow that to happen, least of all our governments. Governments are just as much to blame for this abominable behaviour as the pharmaceutical companies themselves because they are the ones who allow it.

In 2004 the Health Select Committee at Parliament carried out a detailed report entitled 'The Influence of the Pharmaceutical Industry', which was about corruption within the pharmaceutical industry and how the Government played a part in it along with the body that governs them. This was scary stuff to find out but if you have got this far into the book thinking I was fairly normal, and now think that I am an unhinged, tin-foil hat-wearing conspiracy theorist, I urge you to read the report which you can find here http://www.lindalliance.org/pdfs/HofCHealthCommittee.pd. There were hugely important points that the report said would be looked into but, all of a sudden, the work just ceased and one must wonder why – I have my own theories. Another book that can explain what I am talking about is Deadly Medicines and Organised Crime: How Big Pharma Has Corrupted Healthcare, by Peter C Gotzsche. This will give you the real, hard facts to show you that what I am talking about is not nonsense. None of this is conspiracy, it is all proven fact, it is just hidden from the mainstream. The book is written by the co-founder of one of the world's leading medical research institutes so his legitimacy and validity are there to start with. It gives hundreds of examples of corruption within the pharmaceutical industry, right down to specific medications (names included) that were proved to be either more harmful than helpful, or just didn't work. The bit that shook me the most was learning about how pharmaceutical companies modify clinical trials of drugs to work in their favour. This means that the term 'scientifically proven' now holds no standing whatsoever. If trials are modified to suit them, and do not really reflect the truth of the drug, how can we ever trust in anything we are prescribed? The rest of what I am about to tell you will make more sense if you read that book and realise, for a start, that you will not be cured of any illness, disease or ailment by drugs. Fact. If you really think about it, you will notice that there is not one chronic, long-term or terminal illness that has a cure. Chemicals do not heal. Another fact.

So anyway, like I said, that was the first tool, taking my healthcare into my own hands. I realised that there would always be things that doctors would either not pick up on, or not know about and the things that helped me the most were things I figured out on my own, lo and behold, things that didn't involve drugs! Taking healthcare into your own hands is one of the most important parts of this journey for anyone dealing with chronic disease and I urge you more than anything to please think of ways to do this yourself.

The first, most obvious trick is diet. I'd tried things in the past but I had to figure out how to give my body exactly what it needed and what our bodies need are as much whole, real foods as possible and no fake, processed foods. I started juicing every day, mainly vegetables but fruits too and all my food is organic. I have often explained it this way; would you spray toxic ant killer spray on your apple, stick it under the tap for a second then eat it? No, I'm sure you wouldn't. Eating non-organic, chemically grown foods means you are essentially ingesting chemicals with every single mouthful you take. Just like the pharmaceutical industry, the food industry is corrupt. The companies with the most money (likely the ones whose foods have the most addictive, unhealthy ingredients and the most famous slogans) are able to pay their way to the top to ensure that they are marketed and sold relentlessly. You have no idea why you eat the things you have always eaten but they know, they are clever. It's because of this equation: capitalism + commercialism + corruption = most profit. Just like pharmaceuticals, you are brainwashed into thinking certain things are healthy and you eat them every day, such as branded cereals, milk, bread. 80% of what we have been taught is wrong. You will find that the foods that are healthier for you are more expensive because the companies selling them aren't rich and the ingredients cost more because they are natural and it takes more time and effort to produce them. Eating as much fresh fruit and vegetables as possible is important as they have all the nutrients that our bodies need but if they are not organic, we are essentially defeating the object. We wonder why so many people these days get cancer. Just think about it logically: if you made a decision to eat a spoonful of that ant killer every day for your whole life, would you expect to stay healthy? Or would you expect it to cause your body some damage in the long-run? Now I have worded it like that, is it making you think? If you eat non-organic food, this is what you are doing, but the industry has led you to believe it is OK. There is no way we can pump our bodies full of chemicals for our entire lives then expect to be healthy, or wonder why we get ill. If you want to prevent cancer and / or get rid of autoimmune diseases (or any other ailments from allergies to an over-abundance of colds), you have to eat organic.

The foods that are now fashionable to hate: gluten, dairy and sugar. Let's start with sugar. Refined sugar is bad for you, end of, so cutting it out or at least cutting it down as much as possible will be your best bet. But don't listen to these new magazine and newspaper articles telling you to cut out fruit, these are all fads. Our bodies need glucose, fructose and sucrose – from natural sources – so feel free to enjoy fruit. Gluten is the next one; like sugar, it is not great for you. It can inflame the intestines and compromise the immune system and RA, along with probably most chronic diseases, starts and ends with the immune system, which is to do with the gut. So cutting out foods that compromise these is your best bet. Whole wheat foods or gluten free foods are best but don't be fooled by gluten free 'alternatives'. They are just processed foods that don't have gluten. Try things like quinoa and amaranth, and other organic whole foods. Don't be fooled by good marketing schemes that fit the latest fad diet movement. There are plenty of cookbooks and websites with recipes using wholefoods. If I had to pick one out of all these foods to give up, I would without a doubt say dairy. To start with, it is a complete misconception that you NEED dairy for calcium. There is more calcium in a good portion of organic broccoli than in a glass of average cow's milk. Our obsession with dairy is thanks to a range of clever marketing schemes starting in the 1950's encouraging people to drink milk. We are the only species on the planet who still drink milk after infancy, and the only species to think it normal to drink the milk of another species! And it is not necessary, despite what your health visitor or pre-natal care class might tell you about child-rearing. Once the milk has been pasteurised and made suitable for consumption, it loses any goodness it MIGHT have had, and drinking it raw is not an option because of the amount of bacteria it carries. Non-organic dairy cows are injected with the RBGH growth hormone, which is known to cause cancer. This hormone is banned in many countries, but is still used in the US and UK which essentially means we are willingly pumping our bodies full of a cancer-creating chemical in order to consume a product that has absolutely no nutritional value for us. The main reason I stay away from dairy (aside from the chemicals, pus from the cows nipples and the fact that it has no nutritional value for me) is because all the aforementioned issues culminating together mean a decrease in our immune systems. The immune system is essentially housed in the gut and as simple as it sounds (although I bet no doctors ever told you this) the stronger your gut is, the healthier you will be. Dairy kills off a lot of the good bacteria and antibodies in your gut, making way for bad bacteria. This won't just cause stomach problems but a whole range of problems, including autoimmune diseases. After all autoimmune is part of the IMMUNE SYSTEM, so surely, that must be connected to the gut too? If you are reading this and you have arthritis and have had stomach problems for years, I can see a light bulb popping up above your head right about now. Despite what doctors may have told you on the numerous times you've been to have your stomach checked, IT IS CONNECTED. The whole body is connected, this is where modern medicine goes wrong, it doesn't see the body as a whole, it tries to treat individual ailments instead of treating the body but I'll get back to that in a little while. So here you've learned that dairy will not help your gut, which will lead to lower immune system, which will lead to more illness. Moral of the story? Cut out dairy!

To aid your stomach back to health, probiotics are really important. I find probiotics to be one of the things that helped me the most. As soon as my gut got better, my immune system boosted and I started feeling better all round. A good, strong probiotic from a health shop will do the trick.

Our meat is also full of chemicals. Animals are injected with hormones and steroids to make them grow and we are ingesting these cancer and illness-creating chemicals willingly. Organic meat is better, but not completely free of chemicals and although I used to justify eating meat with the fact that kosher meat is killed in a way that doesn't hurt the animal, kosher meat can't be organic, so ethically as well as for health reasons, I don't find that eating meat is best for us or our planet. Although yes, meat contains the essential amino acids we need to rebuild and repair, meat is extremely acid-forming. Humans, unlike meat-eating animals, take days to digest meat because of the acid which means it putrefies on the way through the digestive system, forming waste products that can be toxic to our systems and also causes bloating and indigestion, so we are essentially defeating the object by eating it when we can get protein and amino acids from other, healthier foods. If you want to continue eating meat, ensure that you are buying organic, free-range meat only.

I had constant blood tests because I was always tired. And I'm talking exhaustion beyond comprehension. The kind of tiredness no one could ever imagine until they've gone through it. The blood tests always came back negative, which was a good thing, but what was it that was causing this unrelenting exhaustion? Well, one doctor diagnosed me with Fibromyalgia, which also is common when secondary to autoimmune disease, but to me, it just felt like a name they give something when they don't really know what is wrong. A bit like the IBS in my stomach. I didn't have something with a title of Irritable Bowel Syndrome, and I didn't have something with a title of Fibromyalgia. I had an autoimmune disease and my body was out of balance so all these other things started happening as danger signals.

The blood tests never showed my vitamin B12 levels to be

low, they were supposedly always normal. Eventually, after lots of research, I found out that there was a direct correlation between vitamin B12 and pain. A lack of vitamin B12 in the body affects the nervous system which could cause pain because the nerve endings are too sensitive. Fluoride and the contraceptive pill also reduce vitamin B12 levels so I decided to get a good brand of vitamin B12, get fluoride-free toothpaste, come off the contraceptive pill and stop drinking tap water (our tap water has ridiculous amounts of fluoride in it). Within two weeks my pain levels started to drop, namely, the horrific pain in my jaw that had debilitated me for three years. I learned from this that not everything shows up on blood tests or scans, so we need to listen to our bodies. It turns out that my B12 levels were on the low side of normal, but because they were still in the 'normal' range, no one bothered telling me this. Now, when I have a blood test, I don't bother waiting for the doctor's response, I ask for a print out of the results and check it over myself. I have had to educate myself on the correct and healthy levels for B12, thyroid, iron and many other things and this really is the crux of taking your healthcare into your own hands.

At this point, I began to recognise that the opportunity to get completely healthy was within my reach. I realised that there was so much I didn't know, so much the doctors didn't know, and I was determined to figure it all out for myself, so by eating organic food, juicing, cutting out dairy and having gluten and sugar no more than once a week, taking the probiotics and vitamin B12 along with all the other tips, things started changing drastically.

I had been treated at the Royal London Hospital for Integrated Medicine in Great Ormond Street for a few years by this point and I loved it there. It was previously called the Royal London Homeopathic Hospital but they didn't just offer homeopathy so they changed the name. Dr. Peter Fisher, homeopathic rheumatologist, clinical director of the hospital and physician to the Queen, was my main doctor there. I was also under top homeopathic podiatrist, Dr. Tariq Khan, cognitive behaviour specialist, Dr. Raj Sharma, and acupuncturist and homeopathic physician, Dr. Helmut Roniger. All of these people are fascinating. They are all medically trained doctors who felt something lacking in conventional medicine and decided to go into the field of integrated medicine and I have had wonderful experiences with all of them.

I am now with a private homeopath who also practices Reflexology, Kinesiology, Reiki and Craniosacral Therapy among other things and I've had the best results since being with a practitioner who uses a complete integrated approach to healthcare. She also prescribes supplements along the way.

Fairly recently, I got diagnosed with a gene mutation called MTHFR. MTHFR makes you susceptible to autoimmune disease and also means that the body doesn't absorb things like B12 and folic acid. It could be that when my mum was pregnant with me, the folic acid she took did not reach me as it could not be absorbed and this made me more susceptible to the arthritis. With a low immune system and a body that couldn't absorb certain nutrients and instead converted them into toxins, I was then pumped full of toxins from vaccinations and that was the final call before my body started crying out for help. So really, it is not 'with no defined cause', there is always a reason. Finding out about MTHFR has also been a saviour as I now know what form of B12 and folate to take to ensure that my body gets all the nutrients it needs. This is especially important during pregnancy. It turns out that around 50% of people are walking around with this gene mutation and no one knows it, even the doctors I spoke to knew nothing about it and gave me all the wrong advice. I was lucky I looked into it myself and got in touch with an MTHFR specialist in America so I knew how to treat it and I have now even managed to educate some of my doctors about it. If you can, get the test, it might end up helping you make sense of a lot of the reasons for certain illnesses in your life. It turns out that if you have this MTHFR gene mutation, some medications, including Methotrexate (which is the M I speak about in my book) is totally toxic for you. If doctors are adamant that people need these drugs, surely they should know to check for things like MTHFR. Aside from the fact that the drug is toxic anyway, I may not have gotten as ill as I did if we'd have known about MTHFR back then.

After publishing the first edition of this book, I was asked to become a trustee of the British Homeopathic Association and I am now their youngest ever trustee. During the last four years with the BHA and as patient spokesperson for the Royal London Hospital for Integrated Medicine, I have learned so much. In campaigning to keep homeopathy available in the NHS, we have come across much adversity but we keep on with our plight. The Science and Technology Committee at the House of Lords who claimed that homeopathy was unethical and should not be provided on the NHS are in fact sponsored by a pharmaceutical company, so that takes me back to my original point. Everything is about politics and money and though we have spent our lives believing what we have been told, perhaps now that needs to change. Societies are set up in a way that supports corporations, large earners, not the majority of us. If this wasn't the case then your doctor would let you know that vitamin B17 and hemp oil have cancer killing properties before giving you chemo, that arthritis can be healed by boosting the immune system and strengthening the gut – as can HIV –, that in most cases if you take probiotics you will not be likely to need antibiotics, that cow's milk is, in fact, not what your baby needs and that despite the fact that research isn't always allowed to be published in drug company-sponsored medical journals, homeopathy *does* work.

I'd like to end this section of the book with not an answer per se, but perhaps a vague theory of my own, to a question I'm sure you have been asking yourself since day one if you are reading this because you or your child has been diagnosed with an illness. What causes arthritis? Or any illness for that matter? Well, as we know with the arthritis that I had, 'idiopathic' meant 'no defined cause'. No one ever knows why these things start. Well, no one in the world of modern medicine anyway. In holistic medicine it is the first thing they try to figure out! When one gets diagnosed with cancer, conventional doctors will never ever look to see why or how it started, they just look at trying to remove a tumour and stop it coming back. If someone contracts HIV, it is likely because of an exchange of bloods or bodily fluids but why did that person contract it? We now know that some people have not been infected despite contact with those infected. Why didn't they get it? What stopped them from contracting it? Why did a child get arthritis or autism or ADHD when others didn't? My firm belief is that these things don't just happen because God wills it to. My first point lies within what I mentioned above – immune system. It all begins and ends there. I won't get started with the debate about vaccinations, I'm sure my views on it are apparent by this point in the book, but I will give my theory on how it is connected to illness. Something like JRA would likely be dormant in a child's system from birth, perhaps because of something to do with the mother during pregnancy and that can be anything from a deficiency, something she consumed, low immunity, drugs that were taken (even prescription), stress – anything that could compromise immunity passing through the placenta to the unborn child. This series of events would lead to the child's immune system being pretty low when it is born, but this is not something anyone would know or take notice of. If the child is healthy, he or she is healthy, end of. So if you don't know that something that happened during pregnancy may have caused the baby to have low immunity, you wouldn't know to do things differently, but that low immunity could lead to a dormant disease that may never be triggered if the immune system was built up in the right way, but could easily be triggered by the mammoth strength of vaccinations. In my case, I had the MMR, then got a virus and a few weeks later the swelling appeared in my ankles. My body was screaming out for help. Now, had I not have had the vaccinations that compromised my immunity, and had I not have had any dairy and only eaten organic, chemical free foods, along with doing everything else that could boost immunity, the arthritis may never have been triggered. So what I'm saying here is that vaccinations don't necessarily cause illness (although in some cases I strongly believe they do), but in cases like mine they trigger something that may never have been triggered because they are just too strong for the immune system of a young infant or toddler. So if you're reading this and it's 'too late', you or your child already has an illness, there is no going back in time, but the trick is immune system, even after diagnosis. And if you're reading this and you don't have a sick child (lucky you!) optimum health during pregnancy and immune boosting after birth are key. So I can't change things for you (or for me and my mum!) and take away what has happened, but you can move forward from this with more answers than when you started and a way forward that could see you reach the point that I have reached. I have, after all, seen many people over the years who have followed me into remission with the same tactics.

If you take away any advice from this book, let it be that not everything you are told will be correct, not every doctor knows everything, and you have the tools at your very disposal to change your life and be healthy NOW. You just have to accept that your mind-set needs to change, those misconceptions you have been led to believe your whole life may not be right and you can think for yourself and create a healthier, more fulfilled life. Drugs will not cure. You can do that all by yourself. Now don't you feel empowered? I sure do!

To end on a positive note, not only did the arthritis itself go into complete remission, but the uveitis in my eye also went into remission for the first time ever. When and how? After I came off the steroid eye drops. I started getting pains in my eyes – which the B12 helped a great deal – but it only got completely better once I trialed, for the first time ever, coming off the drops at twenty-nine years of age. Within two months of coming off them – and taking into account all the other natural anti-inflammatory work I'd done along with the right level of homeopathic remedies carefully administered by my homeopath – I was told by Mr. Pavesio that the uveitis no longer showed and for the first time ever, since diagnosis at the age of three, it was in remission. Suffice it to say he called over his whole team to take a look at me. They were in awe.

I have been with not one pain or swollen joint for over two years now.

Staying healthy the natural way isn't easy. It involves a lot of work from pre-preparing meals and juices, to buying produce that isn't available at a local supermarket, to having different treatments and spending time and money on oneself that someone else may not need to do. But it has taught me so much and I am so dedicated to my health and I believe that I am blessed to now have all this amazing knowledge. I now also practice Transcendental Meditation twice a day and do yoga, as well as other exercise. My health is my main priority.

I now dedicate all my time to writing, campaigning and public speaking and I just love the fact that I get to do what I'm passionate about and pass it on to others.

I got married to Daniel in June 2013 on the beach in Israel and I owe him my life. He stuck by me when I was at my very worst and we are now able to enjoy life together now I am at my very best. We live in North West London with our two dogs and we are expecting our first baby in October 2015.

If someone asked me now if I would change anything, I wouldn't. Having arthritis meant that I have gone through things that I wouldn't wish on my worst enemy, but these experiences have shaped and moulded me into a better person. I don't know if I would be as understanding of others if I hadn't have needed so much understanding myself, and I am sure that I would not be so determined to make a success of my life if I didn't know what it feels like to get kicked to the bottom. That determination comes from knowing what life is like without all the good stuff. If I had've been born completely healthy, I would never have strived to be anything more than average. I would not have had the will to succeed and I would not be doing the wonderful things I now do. The only difference between me and other people who have chronic illnesses is that I took it into my own hands and believed there was a way around it, that illness starts for a reason and if we find that reason, we can get rid of it. Cancer or arthritis, psoriasis or diabetes – essentially they are all the same. If you love yourself and treat your mind and soul as well as your body, you can never truly be beaten by disease.

Many people will use their illness as their shield; they believe that they are safe behind their illness. If you hide behind your illness, then you have become your illness. You believe that it makes you who you are. It is not who you are. The best we can do is take the hand that we have been dealt and learn as many lessons from it as possible, so that, one day, we can turn around and say 'my illness contributed to getting me where I wanted to be, but it will never be who I am.' Life will always throw obstacles in our way, but I now believe that life is about how you overcome those obstacles.

The End.

'I just wish I could take away her pain. I feel so helpless and just wish I could make it better,' I heard Mum say on the phone to her friend Jackie as I sat in the kitchen listening intently to her conversation while she stood outside having a cigarette. She ended the phone conversation shortly afterwards and came back into the kitchen where I was sitting, unable to get up due to my last aggressive flare-up. 'You do make it better, Mum. Without you, I wouldn't be where I am today and I wouldn't be able to carry on. You give me strength.' Mum hugged me fiercely and I knew that she was about to cry – until the ever-ringing telephone distracted her.

Through perseverance many people win success out of what seemed destined to be certain failure.

Benjamin Disraeli

Lightning Source UK Ltd.
Milton Keynes UK
UKOW06f1821100615

253247UK00018B/392/P